www.harcourt-interna

D1537074

Bringing you products from all Harcour
companies including Baillière Tindall, Churchill Livingstone,
Mosby and W.B. Saunders

● **Browse** for latest information on new books, journals and
electronic products

● **Search** for information on over 20 000 published titles with
full product information including tables of contents and
sample chapters

● **Keep up to date** with our extensive publishing programme
in your field by registering with eAlert or requesting postal
updates

● **Secure online ordering** with prompt delivery, as well as full
contact details to order by phone, fax or post

● **News** of special features and promotions

If you are based in the following countries, please visit the
country-specific site to receive full details of product
availability and local ordering information

USA: www.harcourthealth.com

Canada: www.harcourtcanada.com

Australia: www.harcourt.com.au

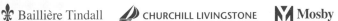
Baillière Tindall CHURCHILL LIVINGSTONE Mosby 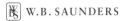W.B. SAUNDERS

Assisting at Podiatric Surgery

For Churchill Livingstone:

Senior Commissioning Editor: Sarena Wolfaard
Project Manager: Gail Wright
Design Direction: Judith Wright

Assisting at Podiatric Surgery

A Guide for Podiatric Surgical Students and Podiatric Theatre Assistants

Telford Thomson
BSc FCPod DPodM MChS SRCh

Holder of the Meritorious Award of the Society of Chiropodists and Podiatrists, awarded in recognition for contribution to the advancement of podiatric surgery within the UK; Fellow of the Surgical Faculty of the College of Podiatrists, UK; Former Tutor in Podiatric Surgery; Private Practitioner, Ipswich, UK

with a contribution from

Denise Freeman
DABPO FACFAOM

Associate Professor of Podiatric Medicine, College of Podiatric Medicine and Surgery, Des Moines University Osteopathic Medical Center, Des Moines, Iowa, USA

Foreword by

Vincent J Mandracchia
DPM MS Board Certified in Foot and Ankle Surgery by the American Board of Podiatric Surgery

Director, Foot and Ankles Clinics; Director, Podiatric Residency Training Program, Broadlawns Medical Center, Des Moines, Iowa; Clinical Professor of Podiatric Medicine, Des Moines University— Osteopathic Medical Center, Des Moines, Iowa; Consulting Editor, *Clinics in Podiatric Medicine and Surgery*, USA

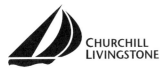

CHURCHILL
LIVINGSTONE

EDINBURGH LONDON NEW YORK PHILADELPHIA ST LOUIS SYDNEY TORONTO 2002

CHURCHILL LIVINGSTONE
An imprint of Harcourt Publishers Limited

© Harcourt Publishers Limited 2002

🖊 is a registered trademark of Harcourt Publishers Limited

The right of Telford Thomson to be identified as author of this work
has been asserted by him in accordance with the Copyright, Designs
and Patents Act 1988

First published 2002

ISBN 0 443 07226 4

British Library Cataloguing in Publication Data
A catalogue record for this book is available from the British Library

Library of Congress Cataloging in Publication Data
A catalog record for this book is available from the Library of
Congress

Note
Medical knowledge is constantly changing. As new information
becomes available, changes in treatment, procedures, equipment and
the use of drugs become necessary. The author, contributor and the
publishers have taken care to ensure that the information given in this
text is accurate and up to date. However, readers are strongly advised
to confirm that the information, especially with regard to drug usage,
complies with the latest legislation and standards of practice.

The
Publisher's
policy is to use
paper manufactured
from sustainable forests

Printed in China by RDC Group Limited

Contents

Foreword

'*A good assistant makes for a good surgeon.*'

I have said those words to my students and residents over the past 25 years because I truly believe them and have witnessed them to be true. The assistant who knows the 'condition of their craft' and anticipates the surgeon is an asset, while one who does not can often be a direct detriment to the procedural outcome. Subsequently, a good assistant becomes a good surgeon.

The practice of podiatry invariably includes surgical procedures, as indeed we are a procedural specialty. Patients who entrust their care to the trained podiatric specialist deserve the utmost care whether undergoing a minor procedure or a major reconstruction of the foot. Paramount to the accomplishment of this optimal care is the podiatrist's ability to fully understand and properly utilize sterile techniques and all other operating room procedures.

Telford Thomson takes the student of podiatry and the operating room assistant through a calculated step-wise approach to patients, including the initial work-up, patient acceptance, procedural protocol and the postoperative care culminating in patient discharge.

No book exists today that covers the basic details encountered in the everyday fulfilment of podiatric procedures and that appropriately prepares the student podiatrist and operating podiatric assistant to properly and expertly perform their duties. Indeed, in my role as an instructor of podiatric medical students, I have not found a single reference book that undertakes and coordinates the task of basic but necessary instruction that allows the podiatrist and assistant to become familiar with proper operating room protocol.

There is nothing more frustrating to a teacher, student or experienced operating room crew than to have a podiatric student or student assistant 'clueless' when entering the surgical arena, the student often citing the lack of available reference material that specifically focuses on the topics of sterile technique and the ability to function as a circulating or 'scrub' assistant.

Telford Thomson freely admits that his text is proscriptive and not prescriptive, but as a reference source of essential basics, it is destined to become a classic. He is to be commended on a fine book; I know that I will certainly encourage my students to be thoroughly familiar with its contents.

Vincent J Mandracchia

Preface

The contents of this book are aimed primarily at the student podiatrist, or non-surgically qualified podiatrist wishing to enter a postgraduate programme in podiatric surgery. Although the principles of sterile technique as explained in this text are equally relevant for the minor nail and skin surgical procedures that are regularly carried out by the majority of today's podiatrists, it is also hoped that podiatry footcare assistants wishing to upgrade to the position of podiatric surgical theatre assistant will find it of some use. Within the United Kingdom, most podiatrists undergoing postgraduate surgical training may well start their practical surgical pupilage first in the role of the surgical assistant and, as they gain experience, progress from circulating assistant to scrub assistant until they are eventually carrying out the surgical procedures as a surgical pupil.

The intention of this book is therefore to take the potential student through the various roles carried out by the assistant from the initial acceptance of the patient as a candidate for outpatient surgery under a local anaesthetic, a form of patient protocol referred to as 'office procedures' by American podiatrists, to the patient's discharge after surgery. This book should not be considered an authority on the anatomy of the foot nor on podiatric surgical procedures.

For convenience, the term 'podiatrist' has been used to refer to a fully qualified podiatric surgeon and the term 'assistant' to refer to podiatric surgical students (who may be fully qualified general podiatrists but who have not undertaken postgraduate training in surgery) or footcare assistants acting in one of the surgical assistant roles. The terms 'operating theatre' and 'operating room' are synonymous and are used interchangeably throughout the text.

While it is difficult to describe accurately the role of the professional podiatric surgical assistant (as opposed to that of the podiatric surgical pupil), as I have found from personal experience that their duties appear to cover everything from changing the water in the goldfish tank to assisting at surgery, nevertheless there is no doubt that the podiatric surgical assistant is a key figure in the successful outcome of many surgical procedures, as well as in the efficient running of the department. It is the experienced assistant's expert working knowledge of the surgical equipment and instruments used in podiatric surgery, as well as the day-to-day management of patients, that makes the podiatric surgical assistant such an asset in the operating room environment.

There are two principal roles for the podiatric surgical assistant in the operating theatre: circulating assistant and scrub assistant. The first can be likened to that of a circulating nurse, sometimes known as the 'dirty nurse' in a hospital operating theatre; the second is that of the scrub nurse. Although both roles are discussed separately, it must be remembered that assisting in the operating theatre is very much a team effort and many of the duties of the circulating and scrub assistant overlap.

It is not my intention to say, 'You must do this my way'; instead, I hope that the contents of this book may give readers some food for thought. You may disagree with some of the points raised and say, 'We don't do it that way.' Why not? All I would say is that the procedures explained in this text have seen me, my patients and staff safely through some thousands of podiatric surgical procedures.

Ipswich 2001   Telford Thomson

Acknowledgements

I would like to express my gratitude to the people who spent some considerable time and effort in reading the manuscript and making some helpful comments for the contents of the various chapters. First among these is my wife, who spent many months reading, correcting and helping to clarify the text for each chapter.

Others are John Malik, consultant podiatric surgeon and tutor at the Birmingham School of Podiatry, for his helpful suggestions and supplying a photo for the cover; Angela Youles of Timesco Surgical and Medical, for providing photographs of surgical instruments; the staff of the Ipswich Hospital NHS Trust Medical Library for their helpful advice whilst searching for suitable material; the Ipswich Hospital NHS Trust Medical Illustrations Department, for providing a number of the photographs that appear in this book; Raymond Mallett, Manager of the Sterilization Department, Ipswich Hospital NHS Trust, for his advice with regard to cleaning and general care of surgical instruments; and Dr Denise Freeman of the College of Podiatric Medicine and Surgery, Des Moines, Iowa, for her suggestions and contributions to the manuscript.

Final thanks go to Dr Vincent J Mandracchia, Clinical Professor of Podiatric Medicine, Des Moines University—Osteopathic Medical Center, Des Moines, Iowa, for taking the time to read the manuscript and for providing the foreword.

1

Patient assessment prior to surgery

THE PREOPERATIVE ASSESSMENT OF THE PATIENT

The initial preoperative assessment of the patient will in most probability be carried out by the podiatrist who is going to undertake the operation. However, there is no reason why an experienced assistant, with the necessary training and qualifications, cannot carry out this assessment.

Although the general principles of the preoperative assessment applies to all forms of podiatric surgery, there will undoubtedly be slight variations in the criteria between different surgical facilities. In addition, this degree of variation will depend to a greater or lesser extent on the individual podiatrist carrying out the surgical procedure.

In most instances the preoperative assessment will normally be broken down into four stages:

1. diagnosis
2. reason for surgery
3. minimum examination (medical)
4. minimum examination (social).

   1. Diagnosis. The initial diagnosis will cover any of the foot pathologies that fall within the scope of practice of the clinic that you are working in.

   2. Reason for surgery. In other words, this describes why the patient wishes to have surgery. Many podiatrists are of the opinion that at least two of the following indicators for surgery must be present to justify an operation:

- pain
- infection
- ulceration
- disability
- bursitis
- painful corn
- inability to wear conventional footwear
- failure to respond to non-surgical treatment
- limited range of movement in the foot or the hallux leading to pain on walking
- in hallux valgus, an overriding or underlapping second toe.

> **TIP:** Justification for surgery is an important consideration, if only to reduce the likelihood of litigation should something unforeseen occur.

When evaluating the patient it is vital that you also take into account the *patient's expectations* with regard to the proposed operation. The patient must also be advised as to any of the possible complications that may occur during or after the operation.

> **TIP:** It may be advisable to have written evidence that the patient was informed of the possible complications, preferably signed by the patient, but separate from the actual surgical consent form.

3. Minimum examination (medical). This should cover such items as:

- blood pressure
- full blood count
- urine for glucose
- adequate pedal pulse
- arterial supply to the legs and foot
- details of current medication and any medication taken within the previous 6 months
- detailed medical history of the patient
- any previous hospital admissions
- family medical history.

> **TIP:** When assessing a patient's medical history, do not take at face value a simple statement on a doctor's referral letter that the patient is suitable for podiatric surgery. It is not unusual for a medical doctor to over- or underestimate the scope of practice or criteria for podiatric outpatient surgery.

4. Minimum examination (social). This should take into consideration the fact that the patient is going to be discharged a short time after surgery, so as well as the medical considerations you must also evaluate the social environment of the patient. This examination should also take into account the patient's age and social background, as both may have some bearing on the postoperative results.

> **TIP:** Patients should be judged on physiological rather than chronological age.

When you are evaluating the patient, answers to the following questions should be sought. If the answer to any of them is in the negative, perhaps you should reconsider whether the patient is a suitable candidate for outpatient surgery:

1. Is someone available to accompany the patient to the department and return the patient home?
2. Is there anyone who can stay with the patient for at least the first 24 hours after surgery?
3. Does the patient have a telephone?
4. Does the patient use any ambulatory aid (e.g. walking stick, crutch, or Zimmer frame), in which case will the patient be able to manage when wearing a postoperative shoe, or plaster cast?
5. Are the living conditions such that the patient can move easily between, say, a bed and toilet?
6. Are the living conditions such that the dressing/wound can be expected to be kept clean and dry?

> **TIP:** Bear in mind that, when patients state that their husband, wife or a friend can look after

them during the early postoperative period, you must consider the possibility that the patient may not be fully aware of the care that may be needed, or overestimate the assistance that a relative or friend can give, especially if that person is elderly.

One question that people often forget to ask is whether the patient has arranged to go on holiday (within the estimated postoperative recovery time).

PRESURGICAL TESTS CARRIED OUT BY SURGICAL ASSISTANTS

As a qualified surgical assistant, or as a podiatry student undergoing surgical training, you will be expected to assist during the presurgical examination of the patient. During this examination you may also have to test the patient's urine, take the patient's blood pressure and on occasions even take blood samples.

Testing urine

Patients presenting for any form of podiatric surgery will normally during their presurgical assessment have their urine tested for glucose as a standard test for diabetes mellitus.

> **TIP:** A surprising number of patients are found to be undiagnosed diabetics.

The urine test can be conducted in various ways but probably the easiest type, and the one that you are most likely to use, is that of reagent strips. Clinistix® are the most common of these.

How to use Clinistix®

1. Collect a fresh urine specimen (if possible use a proper urine collection container).
2. Take a strip from the Clinistix® storage bottle. Check that the expiration date on the bottle has not passed, and that the bottle has not been in use for *longer than 6 months*.

> **TIP:** The date that the bottle was first opened must be entered on the bottle. Failure to do so could result in using out-of-date strips, which may give erroneous readings. If there is no date on the bottle then do not use it.

3. Dip the test area of the strip into the urine and remove immediately.
4. Tap the edge of the strip to remove excess urine.
5. Compare the test area with the colour chart on the bottle *exactly 10 seconds after wetting*.
6. Ignore any colour changes that occur after 10 seconds. *The result is positive if the colour of the test area changes.* You will notice that the colour blocks on the bottle are in differing shades of purple: light, medium and dark. These represent the relative amount of glucose present in the urine.

> **TIP:** If the result is positive do not tell the patient but advise the podiatrist, who may then wish you to take a blood sample.

If the podiatrist requests a blood test to confirm the presence of glucose you should indicate your urine test findings on the blood test request form—for example, as 'urine ++' for a patient with a medium colour change.

Taking blood samples

As well as testing for glucose, blood samples taken prior to podiatric surgery are normally for a full blood count (FBC) or complete blood count (CBC) or, on occasion, urea and electrolytes (U & E).

Depending on local protocols and your training, you may be expected to take the blood samples from patients. At first this may appear to be a daunting challenge, but like everything else practice makes perfect.

Although podiatric surgical pupils learn to take blood samples as part of their surgical training, assistants who are not podiatric students but who are working in or undergoing their training in a teaching unit will normally be shown the technique by one of the unit's tutors. In addition, most hospital haematology departments run a short course for their phlebotomists, and assistants may be expected to undertake this course.

As a student you will not initially be expected to take blood from a known high-risk patient. However, some assistants may be concerned by the dangers of accidentally contracting a blood-borne infection like hepatitis B or the human immunodeficiency virus (HIV). *Therefore when taking blood you should follow the guidelines of your local hospital with regard to the taking of blood samples.*

> **TIP:** Remember that gloves will not protect you from a needle-stick injury, but only from blood spillage and contamination.

Irrespective of the patient's medical category you must be careful. If you wear gloves, dispose of used needles and syringes into the correct containers, and take care when transferring blood from syringes to containers you are at little risk of being infected.

Needle-stick injuries

If you prick your finger with a contaminated needle you should:

1. wash your finger with soap and water and at the same time encourage it to bleed freely
2. swab the wound with spirit or antiseptic and cover it with a sterile dressing
3. note the patient's name and hospital/clinic number; in some hospitals it is policy to obtain a blood specimen from the patient to test for hepatitis B or other infections
4. fill in an accident form and advise the head of your department.

Veins

When you come to take a blood sample, finding a suitable vein is a potential problem. Veins also come in various sizes, each of which presents its own complications.

1. Prominent large veins. These are the easy veins; even if you are inexperienced you are unlikely to miss them.

2. Veins that are deep. These are not so easy. As you cannot see these veins you will have to feel for them, and until you have gained some experience you may find them difficult to locate. Try gently palpating the arm where you would expect the vein to be; you may then feel a slight difference in the density of the skin over the vein. When you think you have found it, run your finger over it to give yourself a picture of where it is before inserting the needle.

> **TIP:** If the vessel is pulsating it is not a vein but an artery.

3. Floating veins. These veins are often found in elderly patients. Although they look easy and fairly prominent they have the frustrating habit of moving away from the needle point as it approaches the vein. You may find that you will have to anchor the vein with your thumb about 4 or 5 cm distal to where you intend to insert the needle. *Once the needle is in place, remove your thumb to release the vein.*

4. Collapsing veins. These veins are normally small and thready and can often bleed after you have withdrawn the needle. *If this should occur advise the patient that bruising may occur.* This problem is often found if you draw the syringe plunger back too quickly as this will cause the vein to collapse and flatten out, stopping the flow of blood. If this happens you should allow the plunger to slide back with the vacuum, then try again.

> **TIP:** To reduce the chance of a vein collapsing draw the blood out slowly but steadily.

5. Very deep-set veins. With obese patients these veins can be very difficult to locate. You should try the normal location, but going deeper than you would normally do. If you have no success *don't give up! Try the back of the hand and if that fails you can always try the foot.*

Taking the blood sample

> **TIP:** First familiarize yourself with the tourniquet you are going to use. You should be able to release the tourniquet using only one hand.

You should also be familiar with the type of syringe and needle that you will be using. (There are various types.) The basic syringe and needle method is as follows.

1. Select the correct needle and syringe, then load the needle on to the syringe, *but do not remove the needle cover.*
2. Place the patient's arm on the arm rest or on a pillow. This stops the patient from pulling back and disengaging the needle.
3. Place the tourniquet around the patient's arm and use it to partly occlude the venous return. The tourniquet is used to make the vein more prominent. It may help if the patient makes a fist or holds a small tube.

> **TIP:** In some cases it is perfectly acceptable to take blood from a prominent vein without using a tourniquet.

4. Locate the vein. *Remember, if it is pulsating then it is an artery.*
5. Clean the insertion site with an alcohol wipe. Remove the needle guard.

> **TIP:** Before inserting the needle into the arm, you should pull back on the syringe plunger to break the seal in the syringe, then return the plunger to its original position (this will make it very much easier to pull back on the plunger when withdrawing the blood).

6. Check that the needle point has the bevelled edge uppermost.

> **TIP:** Do not attempt venepuncture through areas of eczema or sepsis.

7. Slide the needle into the vein, bevel uppermost, along the line of the vein at an angle of about 20° and then withdraw the blood. If no blood is obtained, slowly withdraw the needle while still applying suction as you may have gone through the vein. Blood should be withdrawn at a steady rate, so as not to cause haemolysis. Haemolysis in this case is damage to the red blood cells caused by improper collection, and it could result in an incorrect test result.

> **TIP:** If you do not succeed in obtaining blood after two attempts, you should ask an experienced colleague for assistance.

8. If you are using a tourniquet, release it *before* removing the needle. (This is why you should be able to release the tourniquet using only one hand.) Failure to release the tourniquet first could well result in the formation of a painful bruise.
9. Remove the needle from the vein and cover the puncture site with a piece of cotton wool, asking the patient to press firmly on it.

> **TIP:** Have a cotton wool ball ready in your other hand.

10. Remove the needle from the syringe and discard it into the sharps container. *Do not resheath the needle with the needle cover.*
11. If required, transfer the blood into the correct bottle. (Some syringes double as the bottle, in which case there will be no need to transfer the blood.) Check that you have the patient's name on the sample bottle. If the bottle has an anticoagulant substance mix the blood by gentle inversion.

Bleeding after venepuncture

Occasionally, and often through no fault of your own, there may be bleeding after you have removed the needle. Or there may be bleeding within the tissue during the venepuncture, which will cause a bruise to form. Elderly patients and patients on anticoagulant therapy are more prone to bleeding after venepuncture. The first sign may be that you will see the vein start to swell as you are taking the blood. Release the tourniquet, remove the needle and apply a swab and digital pressure to the area. Hold this pressure until the swelling subsides. Then elevate the arm. If bleeding persists you may well have to hold this pressure for 5 minutes. In some instances you may consider also the application of a tourniquet over the swab for 5 minutes. If one is available, you could apply a cold pack to the area. *It is important to advise the patient that there will be a bruise.*

> **TIP:** The 5 minutes referred to is a measured 5 minutes. When you are holding a pressure dressing this may appear to be a long time. However, avoid the temptation to remove the pressure to see whether the bleeding has stopped before the full 5 minutes have elapsed. The chances are that it will still be bleeding and you will have to start again. This applies equally to a surgical procedure when a pressure dressing is required.

Evacuated system

It is also possible that you will be using what is called the 'evacuated system'. The general principles of this are the same as the above. The difference between the two is that you will not have to transfer the blood from the syringe to a bottle (the syringe in this case is the bottle). Also, the detachable needle has a valve that allows you to interchange the syringes for different blood tests without the need to remove the needle from the vein.

> **TIP:** A point to note is that the colour coding of sample bottles is not universal, as hospitals often introduce their own coding.

Peripheral venous cannulation

In some podiatric departments a part of the presurgical procedure protocol is to insert a venous cannula. The rationale for this is that if a clinical emergency should occur that would require cannulation, for example a cardiac arrest, then the cannula would already be in place, thus saving time.

Various types of cannula are used of which the Venflon® cannula, which has a side port that permits repeated intravenous injections, and the butterfly cannula are both common. The butterfly type is basically a hollow metal needle to which a short flexible plastic tube is attached (this type should if possible be avoided during resuscitation attempts as it can easily become displaced allowing extravasation of administered fluids). The most common form of cannula is a plastic cannula that is mounted on a hollow metal needle, which is used to introduce the cannula into the vein and then removed. The plastic cannula is left in place and secured (Fig. 1.1). You should make yourself familiar with the type used in your department.

> **TIP:** During non-emergency cannulation, until you have gained some experience with venous cannulation you may consider giving a small amount of local anaesthetic just proximal to the proposed point of entry of the cannula.

Technique for inserting the cannula

The principle is similar to that of venepuncture, and the same precautions should be observed. Common sites for peripheral venous cannulation

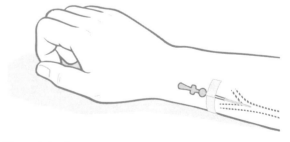

Figure 1.1   A cannula in place (cephalic vein).

are the dorsum of the hand and the cephalic vein at the wrist. The cannula sizes normally used are 18 standard wire gauge (SWG) for saline, and 14 or 16 SWG for blood.

Cannula *if not used* must be flushed at least every 3 to 4 hours and removed after 12 hours. They should also be removed if there is any sign of redness or pain at the insertion site. In all cases the same vein should not be used for longer than 3 days.

Complications that may occur include venous inflammation, thrombosis and sepsis.

Normal reference values in blood tests

> **TIP:** It should be noted that there may be slight variations in values at different hospitals.

As a podiatric surgical assistant you will not be expected to know the different reference values (although surgical pupils will). However, I have found that assistants who know and understand the basic meanings of blood values find that this knowledge gives them a better overall understanding of the podiatrist's responsibilities, as well as adding to their interest in their own role as a surgical assistant. The normal blood values are as follows (see Appendix 1, p. 135, for an explanation of abbreviations):

- Hb (M) 13.5–18.5 g/dl;
       (F) 11.5–15.5 g/dl
- PCV (M) 0.380–0.500 L/L;
        (F) 0.330–0.440 L/L
- MCV 76–96 fl
- MCH 27–32 pg
- RDW 11.5–14.5
- WBC $4–11 \times 10^9/L$
- platelets $135–450 \times 10^9/L$
- reticulocytes 0.2–2.0% ($10–100 \times 10^9/L$).

Differential leucocyte counts (adults)

These are:

- neutrophils $2.0–7.5 \times 10^9/L$
- lymphocytes $1.5–4.0 \times 10^9/L$
- monocytes $0.2–0.8 \times 10^9/L$
- eosinophils $0.04–0.4 \times 10^9/L$
- basophils $< 0.1 \times 10^9/L$.

Plasma viscosities (interpretive guide)

These are:

- 1.50–1.72 normal range
- under 1.50 hypoproteinaemia
- 1.75–2.10 chronic disease states
- 1.72–3.00 acute disease states
- 2.50–3.00 suggestive of myeloma
- above 3.00 suggestive of macroglobulinaemia.

Approximate ranges for some other common blood constituents are as follows (note the values are approximate as the results can vary with the age and sex of the patient):

- urea 2.5–8.5 mmol/L
- Na (sodium) 132–144 mmol/L
- K (potassium) 3.2–5.0 mmol/L
- glucose 3.0–7.8 mmol/L
- creatinine 60–113 mmol/L
- pH 7.35–7.45.

Taking blood pressure

Blood pressure readings should be taken for *all* patients undergoing preoperative surgical investigation.

> **TIP:** It may be prudent to take the patient's blood pressure before taking a blood sample.

Taking blood pressure may appear difficult at first, as you may find difficulty in differentiating the different sounds, particularly if the patient moves and you hear the sound of the tube rubbing against the patient's arm.

Ideally blood pressure readings should be taken with the patient completely relaxed and emotionally at ease. The patient may be seated or reclining, but in either case the arm should be held at the patient's heart level with the arm relaxed and slightly flexed. You can support the arm yourself, or it can be supported on a firm surface (Fig. 1.2).

> **TIP:** If the patient is holding the arm tensely you may get a slightly higher blood pressure reading.

The deflated sphygmomanometer blood pressure cuff is placed around the upper arm, with the centre of the inflatable bladder over the brachial artery. Then, at the same time as you feel the patient's pulse in the wrist (radial artery), you inflate the cuff to a pressure of about 20 to 30 mmHg above the point that you can no longer feel the wrist pulse.

> **TIP:** If you have just taken a blood sample it is advisable to take the blood pressure reading on the other arm.

The stethoscope is then placed lightly over the brachial artery, and the cuff slowly deflated, until you hear the first sound. Note the pressure reading on the sphygmomanometer; this is the *systolic pressure*. Continue to deflate the cuff

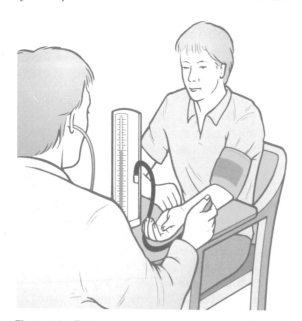

Figure 1.2 Taking the blood pressure, with the patient's arm supported on a firm surface.

until the sounds become faint or inaudible. Again note the pressure; this will be the *diastolic pressure*.

> **TIP:** Some students confuse systolic with diastolic. A way to remember this is to say: 'S for sky which is above'—in other words S is for systolic, which is written above diastolic as in 120/80. It's silly, but it works.

Normal blood-pressure readings

Generally speaking, the average *systolic pressure* in healthy adults under the age of 40 is between: 100 and 140 mmHg.
The *diastolic pressure*
is between: 60 and 90 mmHg.
The average 'norm' is: 120/80 mmHg.

It should be noted that in elderly patients a high systolic blood pressure with a normal diastolic pressure is a frequent occurrence. This is known as *systolic hypertension*, and is a function of the inelasticity of the arteries (arteriosclerosis). For patients over 50 years in age a reading of 150/90 mmHg is considered normal.

> **TIP:** A point to remember is that blood pressure is variable and to some extent depends on age, sex and race. Women normally have slightly higher blood pressure than men, and blood pressure in black people is slightly higher than in white people.

Abnormal blood pressure

A raised diastolic pressure is of much greater importance than a raised systolic pressure. High blood pressure, or hypertension, is when the diastolic pressure reading in adults is over 90 mmHg:

- A diastolic pressure of 95 mmHg is known as *mildly raised hypertension*.
- A diastolic pressure of 105 mmHg is known as *moderate hypertension*.
- A diastolic pressure of 115 mmHg is known as *severe hypertension*.

Patients who are nervous may produce a false reading suggesting hypertension; this is a phenomenon known as *white-coat-induced hypertension*. If you think this is the case you should allow the patient to rest for 10 or 15 minutes and then take the readings again. The second pressure reading will more closely represent the true blood pressure.

> **TIP:** Something you may find is that if three people take a person's blood pressure it is more than possible that you will get three slightly different readings.

Pulse rate

It is desirable to take the pulse rate, normally using the radial artery, in all patients attending for podiatric surgery as it is part of the routine check of the patient's vital signs (i.e. pulse, respiration rate, oral temperature and blood pressure).

As well as taking the radial pulse, you should also check the pulses in the foot (Fig. 1.3), usually the dorsalis pedis (DP) and the tibial posterior (TP). You may in addition wish to test the anterior tibial (AT) pulse to evaluate the general circulation of the foot.

Taking the radial pulse

To take the pulse on the wrist you hold the patient's hand, palm uppermost, and then place three of your fingers—the index, middle and fourth—over the patient's radial artery. Gently compress the artery against the radius.

The slight pressure of your fingers will flatten the artery during diastole, but allow the artery to fill again during ventricular systole.

> **TIP:** Until you are very experienced you should count the pulse for 1 full minute.

The pulse rate will normally be slightly higher in women than in men, with a normal

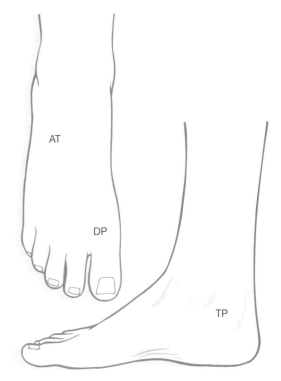

Figure 1.3 Pulses in the foot: the anterior tibial (AT), the dorsalis pedis (DP) and the tibial posterior (TP).

adult rate of between 60 and 90 beats per minute.

In children it can vary with age, the normal values being as follows:

- a child of 3 years of age will have a rate of about 100 beats per minute
- a child of about 7 to 8 years of age will have a rate of about 90 beats per minute
- a young teenager will have a rate of about 80 beats per minute.

It is not uncommon for athletes to have a pulse rate of only 50 beats per minute.

Testing foot pulses for strength and quality

The taking of pulses in the foot assists in evaluating whether any peripheral vascular disease (PVD) is present. The pulses checked are the dorsalis pedis and the tibial posterior, although some podiatrists may also check the anterior tibial artery if they have difficulty in detecting any of the others.

The foot pulses are being palpated for strength and quality, as opposed to rate. They are thus normally registered on a scale from 0 to 4.

When taking the patient's foot pulse with your fingertips if it is found to be 'bounding' this would be registered as a 4. Generally speaking the pulse rate for most patients is found to be 3, which represents a pulse that is good but not as forceful as a 4; this is considered to be satisfactory for all forms of podiatric surgery.

When the pulse rate is registered either a 2 or a 1 the possibility of stenosis or the narrowing of a blood vessel due to a vascular pathology must be a consideration.

If there is no pulse this would be recorded as 0; this may indicate an occlusion that is completely blocking the vessel, although obese patients or patients with severe oedema may also present with a faint or absent pulse.

Doppler ultrasound

All patients presenting for podiatric bone surgery should have their arterial circulation checked by some form of vascular flow detector. This test is commonly referred to as the *ankle/brachial pressure index test*.

> **TIP:** Patients presenting for nail or skin surgery should perhaps also have their circulation checked if they are over 40 years old, smoke or their pulse strength and quality are recorded as below 2.

Ankle/brachial pressure index

As implied by the name the systemic blood pressure is taken at both the brachial artery and at one or all of the ankle arteries. It should be noted that you will *not* be able to obtain a diastolic pressure when using a simple Doppler vascular flow detector. Even though you may have already taken the patient's brachial blood pressure by the standard method of stethoscope and sphygmomanometer, *both* the brachial and the ankle pressure should be tested with the Doppler to *ensure comparability*.

> **TIP:** It is considered a good policy to check the ankle/brachial pressure in any patient who smokes. Smoking can damage the arteries.

Testing

Ideally the patient should have rested for 15 minutes prior to testing. The patient should be supine with the head slightly elevated. Place the cuff around the arm in the normal manner and before inflating the cuff apply a liberal amount of a gel (e.g. K-Y Gel®) to the area where you will place the transducer. Switch the unit on and then with the transducer scan the area until you obtain the best signal. Then gently inflate the cuff until you no longer hear the sound, and take the sphygmomanometer reading at that point; this will be the brachial systolic pressure. (Remember you cannot take the diastolic pressure with a simple transducer.) Compare this systolic reading with the one you took previously by the normal method. If the two are very different you should try again.

Now take the ankle pressure. You will find that in normal subjects the ankle systolic pressure will be higher than the brachial pressure.

> **TIP:** Patients who are non-smokers will often display an ankle pressure of up to 20 mmHg above that of the brachial pressure.

You can calculate the pressure index by the following method:

$$\text{pressure index} = \frac{\text{ankle systolic pressure}}{\text{brachial systolic pressure}}$$

Therefore the normal pressure index will be greater than 1.0. If there is any form of occlusion in a main arterial pathway there will be an abnormal pressure index of less than 1.0.

The pressure index-based criteria for claudication are:

- pressure index > 1.0   normal
- pressure index = 0.05–0.80 one primary arterial occlusion
- pressure index < 0.50   multilevel occlusive disease.

It should also be remembered that, although a number of patients suffering from intermittent claudication may have a normal resting pressure index of > 1.0, it is also possible that after exercise they may have a pressure index of < 1.0.

Intermittent claudication is the name given to the situation when a patient experiences pain or cramping in the calf and leg muscles after walking a short distance, sometimes a matter of only a few yards. The pain is caused by an inadequate supply of blood to the affected muscles.

The transducer

Before using any transducer that you are unfamiliar with you must check the manufacturer's instructions as some transducer heads have to be held at approximately 45° to the skin surface whereas others may be held at 90° to the surface. Having obtained the best sound, hold the transducer steady in position over the artery.

> **TIP:** It may help if you hold the transducer in a way so that the tip of one of your fingers is pressing against the skin, as when the cuff is inflated the patient's arm or leg may rotate, which could cause an unanchored transducer head to move off the artery.

The ideal cuff position when taking the ankle pressure is with the distal edge of the cuff placed just above the malleolus.

> **TIP:** When taking the brachial pressure you may use either the brachial or the radial artery. When taking the foot pressure normally the dorsalis pedis or posterior tibial arteries are used.

X-rays

Whether an X-ray is taken at the preoperative assessment will depend to some extent on the proposed procedure. It is pointless to take an X-ray of the patient's foot just to confirm that the patient has a hallux valgus or some other obvious pathology such as a hammer toe. However, if the proposed procedure is the correction of a hallux valgus deformity, an X-ray can be of considerable assistance in determining what approach the podiatrist should take in the forthcoming operation.

In podiatry X-rays are normally taken to determine whether there is any abnormality in a bone or anatomical structure. The exception to the rule is if the suspected complaint is a neuroma; although this *is not itself visible* on X-ray, a weight-bearing X-ray should be taken to exclude other pathologies such as osteoarthritis, metatarsal stress fractures or osteochondritis of the metatarsal heads.

Something you may like to consider, especially if you are working in a surgical unit where the radiography department is not accustomed to requests from podiatrists, is that when an X-ray of the foot is required the radiographer, unless specifically requested to do otherwise, will in all probability take the film at the previously preset density used for regular foot X-rays. Although this will give a perfectly adequate film of the foot, there will often only be a very poor definition of the toes, especially the distal phalanx. If you wish to have a good film of a distal phalanx to show, for example, a subungual exostosis (Fig. 1.4) you must advise the radiographer to change the settings on the X-ray machine.

Another consideration is that the radiologist who is not familiar with the requirements of the podiatrist will perhaps report a film that to the podiatrist shows a very small exostosis as showing no abnormalities.

> **TIP:** Good communication with the radiography department can save you and your patient a lot of inconvenience.

For most surgical procedures foot X-rays are best taken with the foot bearing weight. The angle that the film is taken from will in most instances depend on the abnormality being examined or the proposed operation. It can sometimes be an advantage to attach a metal pointer to the foot to indicate the location of a foreign body or an area of a soft tissue swelling.

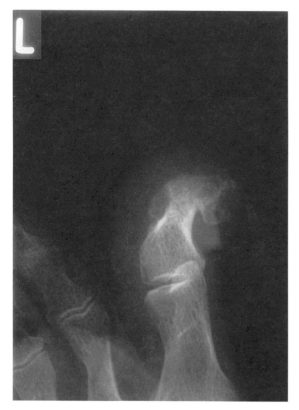

Figure 1.4 X-ray of subungual exostosis. (Reproduced with permission from the Department of Medical Illustration, Ipswich Hospital NHS Trust, Ipswich, UK.)

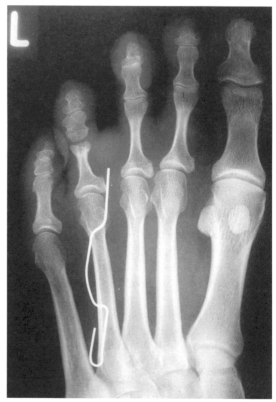

Figure 1.5 X-ray with metal pointer used to show soft tissue swelling. (Reproduced with permission from the Department of Medical Illustration, Ipswich Hospital NHS Trust, Ipswich, UK.)

The metal pointer as shown in Figure 1.5 is used to show a soft tissue swelling. Note the L in the top left corner of this Figure (and in Fig. 1.4); this indicates that it is a film of the left foot. All X-rays should be marked this way to identify the foot and orientate the film (so that you are looking at the foot in the correct sense).

PREPARATION OF THE PATIENT PRIOR TO SURGERY

It is quite probable that some time has elapsed since the patient underwent the initial preoperative examination; if this is the case you should quickly re-evaluate the patient's medical status, paying particular attention to any changes in medication, or hospital admission. When the patient arrives this may appear obvious, but do check first that you have the correct patient and

secondly that all the documentation relates to that patient. For instance, it is possible that you have two Mrs Smiths on the same surgical list.

> **TIP:** Having similarly named patients on the same list is actually bad practice and one that should be avoided if at all possible.

Also, when looking at the X-ray films check that the name and hospital number on the film match the name and number on the transfer envelope. Having confirmed that you have the correct patient and documentation, if the procedure is going to take place in the operating theatre the patient should then change into a theatre gown. A name tag should also be placed on the patient's wrist. Then confirm with the patient that the operation is understood. Finally, the patient must sign the surgical consent form, *before you administer the local anaesthetic.*

In some departments the preparation of the patient's foot takes place with the patient on the transfer trolley. If this is the case the foot should be placed on a waterproof towel and then wiped down with an alcohol wipe prior to any injection. You must also take the patient's blood pressure prior to the administration of the anaesthetic.

> **TIP:** It is recommended that a blood pressure reading is taken for all patients prior to being given a local anaesthetic. The rationale of this is that you will then have a baseline to work from during any emergency situation, for instance if the patient collapses after receiving the local anaesthetic.

Local anaesthetic

As a podiatric surgical assistant you will never be expected to give any form of injectable anaesthetic (unless you are a suitably qualified podiatrist, or surgical student). However, a knowledge of the maximum safe dosage of the two principal anaesthetic agents used may occasionally be of use when you are working as a circulating assistant. For example, a further administration of the anaesthetic may be called for during the operation and if you are logging the amount administered on the count sheet it is your duty to advise the podiatrist if the maximum safe dose is about to be reached. Although it is highly unlikely that the podiatrist would be unaware of this, remember that you are a part of a team and patient safety is of paramount importance.

> **TIP:** Precautions should be observed in any of the following conditions (in other words, unless you are certain in what you are doing do not use local anaesthetics on these patients): shock, heart block, known drug sensitivity, liver disease, epilepsy, impaired respiratory function, pregnant, or taking monoamine oxidase inhibitors (MAOIs). If in any doubt seek the advice of the hospital anaesthetist.

Two principal types of local anaesthetic are used:

- lignocaine 2% (lignocaine hydrochloride), also known as lidocaine or Xylocaine®
- prilocaine 4% (prilocaine hydrochloride) also known as Citanest®.

Maximum safe doses

These are as follows:

- lignocaine 2% without
  vasoconstrictor   3 mg/kg, max. 300 mg
  with vasoconstrictor   7 mg/kg, max. 500 mg
  —toxic plasma level   5 µg/ml
  —threshold dose for
  onset of toxic reactions   7.4 mg/kg
- prilocaine 4%
  without vasoconstrictor   6 mg/kg, max. 400 mg
  with vasoconstrictor   8 mg/kg, max. 600 mg
  —toxic plasma level   5 µg/ml
  —threshold dose for
  onset of toxic reactions   6 mg/kg.

> **TIP:** Students are advised to confirm maximum safe dosage of local anaesthetic, and the amount to use for different procedures, with their tutors or hospital anaesthetists, and to work within the protocol of their own surgical facility.

Average amounts used in podiatric surgery using prilocaine 4% plain

These are as follows:

- ingrowing toe nail avulsion   2 ml
- hammer toe correction   2–3 ml
- bunion correction   5–8 ml
- amputation of toe   3 ml
- excision of interdigital neuroma   4–6 ml.

> **TIP:** Take care with bilateral procedures, for example bunions, as you can easily reach the maximum safe dose.

Other local anaesthetics that may be used in podiatry include amethocaine, bupivacaine, etidocaine, mepivacaine and procaine.

Injection sites that may be used for different conditions are shown in Figures 1.6 and 1.7.

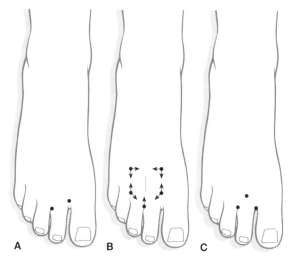

Figure 1.6 Dorsal injection sites. A: Injection sites for hammer toe. B: Injection sites for neuroma ID 2/3. C: Injection sites for digital amputation.

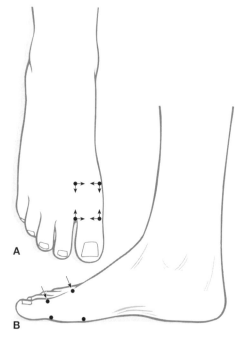

Figure 1.7 Injection sites for bunion procedures (Mayo block). A: Dorsal. B: Medial.

The ankle block

Although all forefoot surgery can be carried out by very localized anaesthesia, some podiatrists prefer to use a method known as the ankle block for regional foot anaesthesia. A number of different areas of the foot can be anaesthetized with this method, depending on which nerves are affected by the local anaesthetic agent.

Some podiatrists dislike this procedure because of the time it can take to obtain total anaesthesia (on average 30 minutes). There is also a danger of penetrating the nerve or adjacent blood vessels, and on these occasions the whole foot may appear to be anaesthetized except for the part you will be working on (not an infrequent occurrence in your early attempts at ankle blocks).

The dorsal nerves of the foot are shown in Figure 1.8. The nerves that can be infiltrated for an ankle block include the following.

The tibial nerve. The tibial nerve (behind the medial malleolus) is infiltrated by the needle being inserted on the medial edge of the Achilles tendon, approximately two finger widths above the centre of the medial malleolus and at right angles to the tibia. You should slowly advance the needle until you can feel the tibia. Then you must aspirate the syringe to ensure you have not entered a blood vessel before you inject the anaesthetic agent.

The sural nerve. The needle is inserted just above and behind the tip of the lateral malleolus and lateral to the Achilles tendon. Then, taking care to miss the small saphenous vein, direct the needle towards (but not touching) the peroneus longus tendon. As above, aspirate before injecting the anaesthetic.

Saphenous and superficial peroneal nerves. Both of these nerves can be infiltrated at the point where they approach the dorsum of the foot between the medial and lateral malleoli. To do this, insert the needle in front of the medial malleolus and then direct it transversely and subcutaneously towards the lateral malleolus. The needle must be kept deep to the superficial veins but superficial to the extensor tendons. As with all ankle nerve blocks, you must aspirate

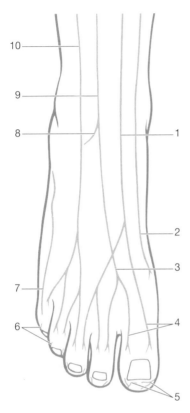

Figure 1.8 Dorsal nerves of the foot.

1. Medial branch of the superficial peroneal nerve.
2. Saphenous nerve.
3. Medial terminal branch of the deep peroneal nerve.
4. Dorsal digital nerve.
5. Medial plantar nerve.
6. Lateral plantar nerve.
7. Sural nerve.
8. Lateral terminal branch of the deep peroneal nerve.
9. Deep peroneal nerve.
10. Lateral branch of the superficial peroneal nerve.

the syringe before you inject, in case you have penetrated any of the superficial veins.

Deep peroneal nerve. This nerve can be infiltrated in the middle of the tarsus, where it lies between the extensor hallucis longus tendon and the extensor digitorum longus of the second toe. To do this, insert needle at right angles to the dorsum of the foot, between the extensor tendons but lateral to the dorsalis pedis artery. (You must feel for this artery before inserting the needle.)

The principal complication of this procedure is accidental penetration of the nerve with the needle. This can lead to long-term pain for the patient.

Apex of the toe. If a procedure is to be carried out on the apex of a toe, for example a fish-mouth incision (Fig. 1.9) for the removal of a subungual exostosis, you should consider that the tips of the toes, as well as being supplied by the dorsal digital nerves, are also supplied by the digital branches of the medial and lateral plantar nerves.

Dermatomes. In considering which skin areas are supplied by which nerves, you should also take account of the dermatomes. A dermatome is an area of the skin that is supplied by any one spinal nerve. The dermatomes of the lower limbs are shown in Figure 1.10. Areas are prefixed by T, L or S, which relate to the spinal nerves; those prefixed with T originate in the thoracic region, those with L in the lumbar region and those with S in the sacral region of the spine.

You will see from the figure that both the sole and dorsum of the foot are supplied by L5 and S1, and that the space between the first and second toes (deep peroneal nerve) is supplied by L4 and L5.

Adverse reactions to local anaesthetics

Overdosage may cause the following central nervous system (CNS) reactions: numbness of the tongue, lightheadedness, dizziness, blurred vision, tremors followed by drowsiness, convulsions, unconsciousness and possibly respiratory arrest.

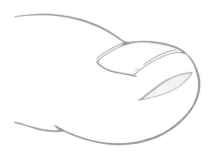

Figure 1.9 Fish-mouth incision.

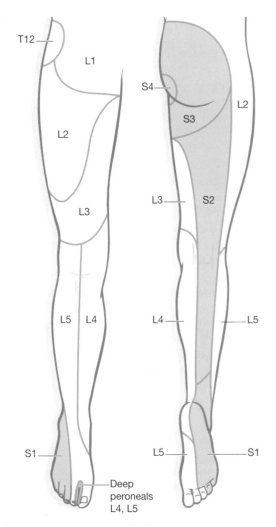

Figure 1.10 Dermatomes in the leg.

Cardiovascular reactions of overdosage include hypotension and myocardial depression.

However, probably the most frequent emergency encountered in the podiatric department is that of the patient fainting after receiving the injection.

Syncope (fainting)

Your first experience of this can be quite frightening as it may occur with no warning at all from the patient. This is why it is important to take the patient's blood pressure prior to administering the local anaesthetic.

In many instances, though, patients state that they feel unwell or giddy. They may then become pale, and sweat may be observed on the face. If this occurs you should lie the patient down with the legs elevated if supine, or place the head between the knees if the patient is sitting.

If the patient is supine and unconscious, maintain an open airway. Loosen all tight clothing. *Call for assistance.* Administer oxygen if available. Loss of consciousness can vary in duration and depth; the patient may also experience a tremor or a clonic jerk (caused by a reduction of oxygen going to the brain). This will be accompanied by a reduction in blood pressure, and a thin or impalpable pulse.

There is frequently a quick recovery after the patient lies down, however, in which case you may not have time to observe these vital signs. Recovery is most often quick, with the pulse increasing and the blood pressure returning to 'normal'.

> **TIP:** After the anaesthetic has been administered the patient must not be left unattended.

Preparation of the foot

Assuming that all has gone well, you will now have to prepare the patient's foot. The foot to be operated on must first be placed on a clean waterproof towel (the foot that is not going to be operated on is placed under this towel). Then, wearing gloves, you should wash the foot with an antiseptic cleaning agent, often povidone–iodine (Betadine®). This preoperative wash removes bacteria and dirt from the skin surface, and also gives an antiseptic cover to the skin surface. When washing the foot you must take particular care to clean between the toes. The foot should be washed at least as far up as the ankle. How far up the leg you then wash will depend largely on the preoperative protocol of the particular unit you are working in.

After the wash, all of the povidone–iodine must be cleaned from the foot with sterile water, then dried using a fresh sterile towel. Note that the skin should be dabbed dry, not wiped.

For some operations the podiatrist may wish you to mark the operation site with a sterile skin pen. Before applying this marker you must confirm the location by checking the preoperative notes and the consent form. This is particularly important if the condition to be operated on is not very obvious—for instance a soft tissue lesion. *There can be no excuse for operating on the wrong foot or toe.*

> **TIP:** You should mark any non-obvious soft tissue lesion, for example a ganglion, with the marker before administering the anaesthetic. This is because the anaesthetic will often swell the tissue around the lesion, making it subsequently almost impossible to locate the lesion accurately.

After the foot is prepared *enclose it* with a fresh sterile towel and fasten this towel in place with a strip of sticking plaster. If required, a tourniquet can now be placed in position approximately 2 cm above the malleolus.

> **TIP:** Cover the tourniquet with an adhesive-edged waterproof towel, fastening the distal edge of the towel around the ankle. This will avoid any splashing of the tourniquet—for instance with preoperative antiseptic paint, which may be applied to the foot in the operating theatre.

Transfer to the theatre

Whilst the patient is waiting to be taken to the theatre, you must ensure that the sides of the transfer trolley are in the up position. Also, do not leave the patient alone at any time.

When you are ready to take the patient to the theatre, check that you have the correct notes, consent form and X-ray films. Remember also that the temperature may be low in the corridor between the preparation room and theatre, so cover the patient with a blanket. This blanket will normally be removed at the theatre door and replaced by another by the theatre staff.

> **TIP:** For procedures carried out under a local anaesthetic, it may be advisable for patients who are asthmatic or have a history of angina pectoris to take their medication into the theatre with them.

2

In the operating theatre

THE ROLE OF THE CIRCULATING ASSISTANT

Although some people may consider the scrub assistant to have the more glamorous role, many others justifiably feel that the role of the professional circulating assistant is far more demanding, as it requires a wealth of knowledge of the various podiatric surgical procedures and theatre protocol, together with a comprehensive understanding of all the equipment used within the podiatric department. This needs to be to a standard far in excess of that required by a new podiatric surgical pupil.

As a circulating assistant, in addition to having to familiarize yourself with the layout of the operating theatre, sterile store and scrub area, you will also have to know the location of any equipment that is normally stored outside the operating theatre. The locations of the defibrillator and extra oxygen bottles are examples. You will also need to know where to obtain any of the extra instruments, sutures, dressings and other equipment that may be required during, before or after the operation. If this was not enough, you will be expected to be conversant with all the paperwork that accompanies the patient into and out of the operating theatre.

Inside the operating theatre as a circulating assistant you will have to be both familiar with and capable of checking and operating all of the theatre equipment—the lights, medical suction equipment, diathermy equipment, systems for maintaining the room temperature and ventilation, the operating table adjustment and the mobile medical gas bottles, to name but a few.

OPERATING THEATRE CLOTHING

Before entering the operating theatre you must consider both general hygiene and the clothing that you will be wearing in the theatre.

> **TIP:** All staff who are employed in the theatre should be free from transmissible bacterial infections. The following conditions are of concern: skin infections such as furuncles (boils), dermatitis, eczema, unhealed wounds and upper respiratory tract infections.
> Staff who exhibit any of these should be excluded from the theatre until they are clear from any infection.

Although theatre staff should have a shower or bath daily you should take this a few hours before you change into your theatre clothing; this is because shedding of skin microorganisms is highest just after bathing. You should, in addition, wash your hands both before and after contact with the patient, and also after touching any item that falls on the floor or any other potentially contaminated surface.

Your head hair (including a beard) is a potential source of bacterial infection. It should therefore be covered at all times by any staff present either in the operating theatre or in any other (clean) restricted area of a surgical suite.

> **TIP:** Surgical head gear should be put on before dressing into a theatre scrub suit; this will prevent hair or dandruff falling on to the scrub suit.

Some considerations about scrub suits

Male and female scrub suits are shown in Figure 2.1. For both versions, the sleeves of the top must be short enough to allow you to wash above your

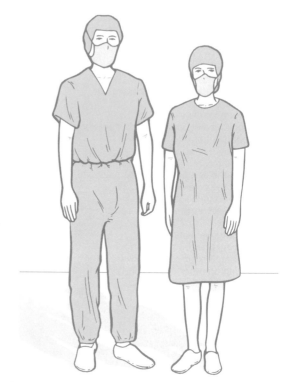

Figure 2.1 Male and female scrub suits (theatre greens).

elbow when scrubbing up. When in theatre, the top of the scrub suit should be tucked inside the trousers. This prevents it swinging and accidentally touching sterile surfaces, and reduces the chance of shedding skin particles on to a sterile surface. The trousers should be closed at the ankles. Female staff wearing scrub dresses should also wear tights to contain any bacterial shedding.

> **TIP:** When putting on scrub trousers take care not to drag the trouser legs on the floor (that is where most of the bacteria are).

Surgical footwear is always a potential source of cross-contamination, so these must never be worn outside the surgical suite. Ideally, you should use disposable waterproof shoe covers and change these after *each* procedure.

If you wear a surgical mask, dispose of this after each procedure as it can harbour bacteria. *When removing masks you should handle only the tie-cords.*

YOUR FIRST DAY IN THE OPERATING THEATRE

There is a lot for you to know and understand and it cannot be learnt quickly. As a new circulating assistant you may feel completely lost, and indeed even frightened at the prospect of entering an operating theatre.

Some new assistants are fearful of humiliation should they faint when observing an operation—a fear that has regretfully been known to deter a number of people from applying for the job. Contrary to popular belief, however, you are most likely to faint if you have been standing on one spot for a long time and not, as you may have thought, from the sight of blood.

> **TIP:** Fainting can often be avoided by having a good breakfast and moving your feet or position while you are observing the operation.

Should you start to feel faint, just walk away from the operating table and sit down with your head between your knees. This applies even if you are 'scrubbed up'; it is far better that the podiatrist finds him or herself suddenly busier than that you faint and fall against the operating table or surgeon.

If you do faint then you will probably find that no one will think you a fool, even though you may have to put up with some banter afterwards. You can take comfort from the knowledge that even some of the surgical staff may well have fainted at some time.

If you are new to the department and it is your first experience of surgery, it is perfectly acceptable to ask the trained assistants whether you may begin by just observing their work during the first part of the day, and then perhaps as the day progresses becoming gradually more and more involved. In a well-run department no one will object, and you can learn a lot by just sitting back and watching. Don't be frightened to stand near the operating table to watch the operation; do get near, as you will not see much from the door.

> **TIP:** Just remember if something is green, or sometimes grey or even blue, do not touch it.

Do not be afraid either to ask the podiatrist questions; most will be pleased to explain things to you. If you have not chosen a good moment to ask then the scrub assistant will soon tell you.

After or between operations the trained staff may well ask you to help in tidying up, or to assist in setting up new trolleys for the next operation. You will soon notice that there is a considerable amount of work to be carried out after the operation. By watching and assisting wherever possible you will learn a lot, making your first few days both an exciting and an enjoyable experience.

Although it is almost impossible to describe completely the role of the circulating assistant, it is probably safe to say that any operation that has been carried out without fuss, complications or delays owes as much of its success to the actions of a skilled circulating assistant as it does to those of the podiatrist.

WORKING IN THE THEATRE: BEFORE THE OPERATION

As in most things, preparation is the secret of success.

> **TIP:** If the operation is the first of the day, this advice may seem obvious, but do check that you are in the correct operating theatre. There is nothing more frustrating to yourself, never mind the inevitable delay caused to the operating list, than spending an hour setting up the wrong theatre.

Equipment check

The first thing you should check is that all of the electrical equipment is safe and in working order. This check should include the theatre temperature and ventilation systems for regulating heat and humidity. If the theatre air-change system works only when the automatic door locking system is operating, this must also be tested.

You should also include in your check: the main theatre ceiling lights, the operating lights, the X-ray viewing boxes and also the emergency telephone, if one is fitted.

> **TIP:** Most items will have a date stamp on them, showing when they are due to be checked or serviced by the appropriate department. (Is it out of date?)

After you have checked all of the fixed equipment and systems to your satisfaction, it is time to turn your attention to the portable equipment. Start with the resuscitation trolley. First, check whether it is in the correct place. Secondly, you must also confirm that none of the drugs are out of date. Thirdly, ascertain that the mobile equipment that is normally to be found on the trolley is present.

In some podiatric departments the responsibility of seeing that the resuscitation trolley is correctly stocked may have been allocated to a particular staff member. Nevertheless it is still a good policy to check the trolley at the beginning of the day. When an emergency situation arises it is not the time to discover that some vital item of equipment is missing.

> **TIP:** Some podiatric surgical units employ a check-list, with a tick-off column of all the items to be checked or tested before the first operation of the day. Don't be embarrassed to make use of it.

If the department carries out its own sterilization of instruments then you should also make sure that the autoclave is in working order and that the water chamber contains the correct level of water.

Within the theatre you need to check that the diathermy switches are working in the correct sequence and that the lead to the foot control is long enough and undamaged.

If fluid suction equipment is employed in the theatre then check that this apparatus is operating correctly. You can do this by switching it on, then putting a finger over the end of the suction tube and seeing that the suction pressure reading increases on the gauge. Then ensure that a fresh tube and extra sterile nozzles are available.

If patient-monitoring equipment is to be used you must check that this is in place and also that it is in working order.

The operating table must also be tested. Check that it moves in all of its planes. If the operating table is mobile, ensure that it is correctly placed under the operating light and that the *brakes are on!*

Checking and changing gas containers

It is your responsibility to ensure that there is sufficient gas in all the relevant containers for the operation. If air-power surgical equipment is to be used, you should also check the contents of the air bottle. Ascertain whether there will be enough, or whether you will have to change the bottle.

Opening and closing gas cylinders

> **CAUTION: Never** use any oil or other lubricant on any cylinder valve or regulator. To do so may cause an explosion. If the valve is stuck then do not use the cylinder; replace it!

Opening a gas cylinder

1. Make sure that all valves are in the 'off' position.
2. Open the main valve (the valve that is a part of the cylinder) anticlockwise (a valve key is normally attached to the cylinder and this key should fit *all* valves). Notice what the reading is on the gauge, if one is fitted. If it is low, the bottle may have to be changed.
3. If satisfactory, open the main valve all the way, then back a quarter turn.

Closing a gas cylinder

1. Check the contents and if they are low then change the bottle.
2. Close the main valve (the one on the cylinder) clockwise.

3. Allow the gas to escape from the system regulator (the gauge that is attached to the main valve).
4. Turn the regulator valve to the 'off' position.

How to change gas cylinders

1. Turn off the gas at the main valve (the valve that is a part of the cylinder) then bleed the regulator (the removable valve that is fitted to the cylinder, and normally has the contents gauge on it).
2. Remove the regulator.
3. Replace the old cylinder with a new one.
4. Remove the protective valve cover on the new cylinder. Then, before fitting the regulator, open and *quickly close* the main valve; this will blow any dust from the valve.
5. Replace the regulator on to the main valve.
6. Open the main valve and check that you get a reading on the regulator. If there is an adequate reading then close the main valve.

Medical gas cylinders used in podiatric surgery

The medical gases most commonly used in podiatry surgery are listed below. All bottles in British medical establishments are identified by colour codes that are *British Standard*, not an international colour code.

As well as colour coding, most medical gas bottles/cylinders use a *pin-index system* (Fig. 2.2) as a further safety feature. In this system, where the gas cylinder attaches to a regulator or anaesthetic machine, there are a number of metal pins. Each gas has a different pin configuration; this makes it impossible to fit a cylinder to an outlet other than its own.

Air. This is used for air-driven surgical saws, K-wire drivers and osteotomes. The bottle size will generally be a 'G'. This bottle is painted grey, with black-and-white quartering at the valve end (with a 'bullnose' valve).

Oxygen. This is used for clinical emergencies. The bottle size may be a 'D', 'E' or 'F'. The bottle is black with a white segment at the valve end (size 'F' bullnose valve, 'E' and 'D' pin-index valve).

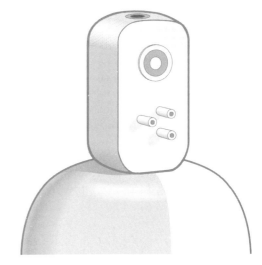

Figure 2.2   A pin-index system.

Entonox. This is used as a mild anaesthetic agent. The bottle size is normally 'F' although a 'D' size, which is portable, may also be used. The bottle is blue with blue-and-white quartering at the valve end (pin index).

Nitrous oxide. This is used in cryosurgery to freeze tissue. The bottle size is 'E', and the colour is blue overall (pin index).

Carbon dioxide.   This is used to inflate automatic tourniquets. The bottle size used on the tourniquet is normally 'C', and the colour of the bottle is grey (pin index).

This is also a good time to check that the carbon dioxide bottle on the automatic tourniquet is full, and to run through the test routine. Remember to *turn off* the gas after testing.

The oxygen bottle on the operating table should also be tested at this time, making sure that a mask and line are fitted and in place.

> **TIP:** Ensure that the keys for the oxygen and air bottle are located near to, or attached to, the bottles.

Instrument check

Once all of the mechanical equipment has been checked it is time for you to consider whether any additional equipment or instruments may be required for the forthcoming operation. (A glance at the operating list will tell you the operations planned for that day.) For example, if a neuroma operation is to be performed then a special metatarsal spreader, which may be a Weitlander self-retaining retractor (Fig. 2.3) or similar retractor, will be required.

You will soon discover that some podiatrists have their own preferences for special instruments, and lists of these instruments are normally to be found in the sterile store, under that podiatrist's name.

The scrub area

When you have finished checking the theatre, turn your attention to the scrub area. Here you should ensure that there are a sufficient number of gowns laid out for the surgical team and that the sterile surgical gloves are of the correct size (the gowns and gloves will still be in their packs, unopened). Ascertain also whether the soap and sterile brush dispensers are full and working.

By checking the operating list you may be able to see whether any specimen jars are required.

> **TIP:** Words like biopsy or excision are the clue.

You will not normally be required to clean the floor or the permanently fixed equipment yourself, as this should have been carried out by the theatre cleaning staff. However, you should just make sure that none of the surfaces or equipment are dirty, wet or stained.

Cleaning

Sometimes, however, you may have to clean the theatre between operations. Exactly how much you will have to do will depend to a certain extent on the protocol of the unit and the procedure that was performed. The following is a list of the basic procedure.

- Wear disposable gloves.
- Brooms or dry dusters should not be used in the theatre or any part of the surgical suite, because they cause air disturbance when used.
- If you use a mop change its head daily (for a freshly laundered one). Use a different head in each room.
- Buckets should also be cleaned between rooms.
- Horizontal surfaces should be damp-cleaned with a detergent germicide.
- Clean off any splashes on doors or walls.
- Surgical lamps should be cleaned only *after* they have cooled.

> **TIP:** Some detergents may leave a film on the lamp, which will reduce or distort the light. Follow the manufacturer's instructions.

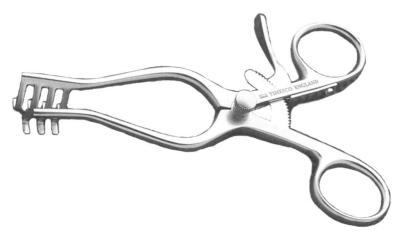

Figure 2.3 Weitlander self-retaining retractor. (Reproduced with permission from Timesco Surgical & Medical, London, UK.)

- When you clean an operating table that has a split mattress (Fig. 2.4), you must wipe each surface separately as debris tends to accumulate between the individual mattress sections.
- All the equipment that does not have to be sterilized should still be cleaned and made ready for the next procedure.
- The floor should be wetted with a detergent germicide before moving the operating table and other equipment. After moving them, you can then mop the floor.

> **TIP:** If you wet the floor before moving the operating table, you will disinfect the castors as they are moved through the detergent.

- All disposable rubbish should be placed in appropriately marked bags and removed from the theatre.

After the theatre is cleaned, and if required for the next operation, you can now place a (clean) non-sterile operating table cover over the operating table; this is often a white draw-sheet. The pillow may also be put in place at this time.

Before the scrub assistant arrives you would ideally have located within the sterile store the instrument packs that will be required for the forthcoming operation.

You should put a face mask on before opening the outer covering of the instrument pack. Instrument packs are normally double wrapped, and you must check that the outer cover of the pack has not been opened or torn. If it has, that pack must be considered to be unsterile and *must not be used*.

> **TIP:** Note that in some instances and in some theatres where only skin or nail procedures are carried out, masks are not worn. This practice will depend on the protocol of the unit you are working in and it is not a national standard. It is bad practice to have your mask hanging around your neck (as seen on TV). Don't do it!

When the scrub assistant arrives

A word of warning: the 'scrub assistant' may turn out to be a surgical pupil with little or no actual experience in an operating theatre, or even a podiatrist, both of whom will find more ways of becoming 'unsterile' than you would have thought possible. Should you observe this happening *it is your duty* to tell the person, and demand if necessary that he or she changes

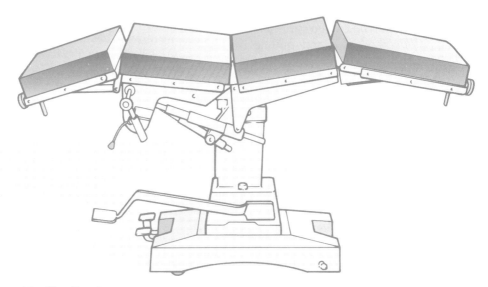

Figure 2.4 Operating table with split mattress.

gloves and regowns. If necessary, replace the complete instrument trolley. Do not allow yourself to be intimidated; no one will criticize you for ensuring that the surgical area is sterile.

After the scrub nurse or other members of the surgical team have 'scrubbed up', one of your duties as a circulating assistant may be to help the surgical team get into their surgical gowns.

Gowning and gloving

You should open the gown pack on a sterile surface. The gown should be folded in such a way that the scrub assistant can touch only the inside of the gown. The neck ties on the gown should be visible.

Gowning with help from the circulating assistant. The procedure is as follows.

1. The scrub assistant, standing back from the sterile surface by about 30 cm, lifts the gown upwards from the sterile surface.
2. Then, holding the gown by the neck ties, the scrub nurse allows the gown to unfold with the inside of the gown towards the wearer, taking care not to touch the front of the gown (Fig. 2.5A).
3. The hands are now slipped into the arm holes (Fig. 2.5B).
4. While holding the hands at shoulder level and away from the body, you can then help by reaching inside the gown and pulling on the inside tags. This will pull the gown up the arms (Fig. 2.5C).

> **TIP:** When the closed glove method (see Ch. 3, p. 42) is employed the gown is pulled up, leaving the sleeve cuff extending over the hand by approximately 2 cm.

5. The circulating assistant can now tie the gown at the neck and inner waist ties (Fig. 2.5D). *The circulating assistant must touch only the inside of the gown.*
6. When a wraparound gown (orthopaedic gown) is used it is only *after* the scrub assistant has gloved that the front ties of the gown can be

untied to allow the gown to be wrapped around to cover the person's back. This is done by the following method: disposable gowns often have one of the front tie ends attached to a paper tag, which the scrub assistant passes to the circulating assistant, and can safely hold this tag without contaminating the gown (Fig. 2.5E). The scrub nurse then turns to the left, while you stand still but continue to hold the paper tag; this closes the gown. The scrub nurse holds the sterile tie as *you* pull off the tag. The scrub nurse then ties the gown at the front (Fig. 2.5F).

The scrub assistant's trolley

Whilst the surgical team is 'scrubbing up' you can start to prepare the scrub assistant's trolley. You will have brought this into the theatre from the sterile store, with the instrument packs on it, still protected by the inner wrapper.

> **TIP:** You should remove the outer wrapper outside the operating theatre (in the sterile store) as it is considered a dust cover, and must not be taken into the theatre.

The inner wrapper, which is normally made of white waterproof paper, is now the new outer wrapper. However, although it was previously 'sterile' it is now generally considered to be only 'clean' as it has been placed on the non-sterile surface of the trolley. This inner wrapper is not to be opened until the trolley is inside the theatre, and the scrub assistant must not touch this wrapper with the surgical gloves.

> **TIP:** Before you open any of the instrument packs, you must check with the scrub assistant that the operation list has not been changed, or that a different instrument pack is required.

It is your task as the circulating assistant to open the inner wrapper (Fig. 2.6). However, before doing so you should make sure that the sterilization indicator strips (Fig. 2.6A) have not

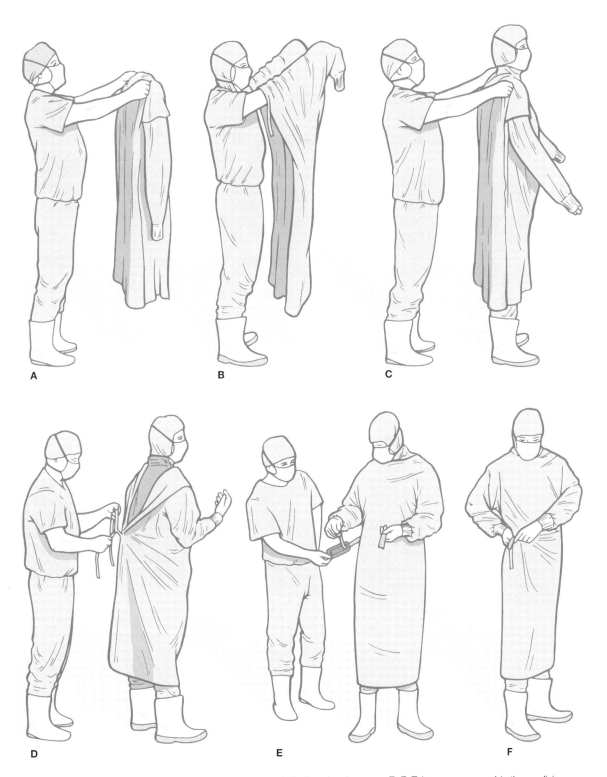

Figure 2.5 Gowning with help from the circulating assistant. A–D: Donning the gown. E, F: Tying a wraparound (orthopaedic) gown.

been torn, nor have changed colour. If either of these is the case you *must not* use that pack.

> **TIP:** If you are wearing a scrub suit, it is a good idea to have the bottom of its top tucked into the trouser tops. This will avoid the possibility of the bottom of the top brushing against a sterile surface.

When opening the inner paper wrapper you must handle only the corners of the paper. You should be facing the trolley, with the pack positioned so the opening fold is facing towards you. Then taking the corners of the paper, open the top fold first and fold it back *away from yourself,* leaving the lower fold in place (Fig. 2.6B). This will ensure that should you lean over the pack you will not touch the sterile green wrapped inner pack, nor drop anything on to it. Then open the side folds (Fig. 2.6C). Now you can unfold the lower fold, this time *towards yourself,* exposing the green sterile instrument pack (Fig. 2.6D).

> **TIP:** Do not touch the inner packing, otherwise you will have to change the pack.

When the patient arrives

Podiatric surgery is usually performed with the patient having received only a local anesthetic; therefore the person will be awake during the procedure, and possibly nervous or anxious. To assist in reducing such anxiety, the patient may be accompanied by another podiatric assistant, who will stay with the person during the operation. This is a task often given to new assistants during their first few days in the department, and on occasions these assistants may also be asked if they could act as a 'second' circulating assistant.

If the patient is a child, it is often hospital policy to allow a parent to stay with the child in the theatre, during the operation. (A parent staying in the theatre with a patient must also wear theatre greens.) Other frequently employed methods to help reduce patients' anxiety may be playing soft music and placing a screen in such a way that patients cannot see their feet.

Transferring and checking the patient

If the patient is transported on a trolley from the preparation room (preop) to the operating theatre by staff who are not wearing theatre clothing, you will have to take over the trolley from them at the theatre door. If there is a blanket over the patient this should be removed before entering the theatre, and possibly replaced by a freshly laundered blanket.

> **TIP:** Whenever a patient is on the trolley, the safety rails on the sides of the trolley must be in the 'up' position.

After taking the trolley from the porter, you should place it next to the operating table. Most importantly, *do not forget to put the trolley's brakes on before you lower its safety rail* on the side nearest the operating table so that the patient can be transferred from the trolley to the operating table. If you fail to do this, the patient could easily fall between the trolley and operating table, if the trolley moves.

> **TIP:** When you take the paperwork and X-rays accompanying the patient into the operating theatre, check that this paperwork actually refers to the patient on the operating table, and that the consent form has been signed.

After you have safely transferred the patient on to the table, make sure that the person's feet are the correct distance from the end of the table (about 25 cm). This is so that the podiatrist is able to reach the patient's feet without having to stretch, and this is especially important when dealing with short patients (and equally for short podiatrists).

> **TIP:** When the patient arrives in the theatre, check that the person is not wearing

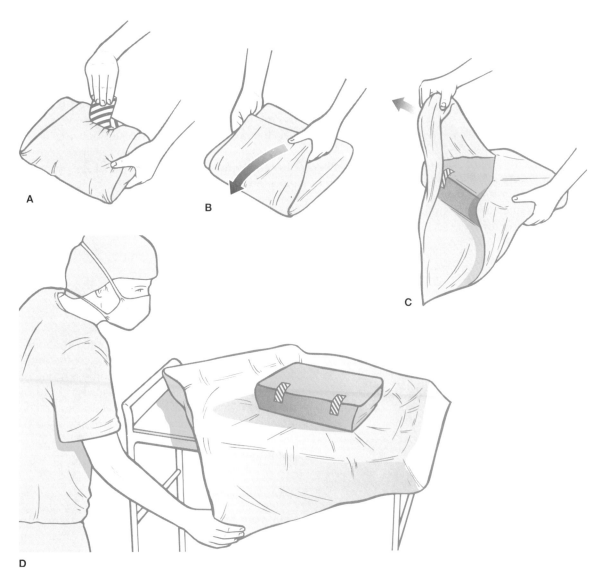

Figure 2.6 Procedure for opening the wrapper of an instrument pack. A: Check sterilization indicator. B: Open the first fold away from yourself. C Open the side folds. D: Open the lower fold towards yourself.

a metal necklace or bracelet, as there is the small possibility that these could cause a skin burn if diathermy is used. Wedding rings should be covered with tape. If the patient is wearing lipstick this should also be removed as it could disguise any colour change that may occur during a clinical emergency.

Attaching and arranging equipment

Before the surgical team places the sterile green drapes over the patient, you should attach to the patient any instruments or monitoring equipment that is required for the operation. This may include the tourniquet cuff, although in some departments the cuff is fitted to the patient's ankle in the preop room before the patient arrives in the theatre.

> **TIP:** When attaching the lead of the pulse-oximeter (Fig. 2.7) to the patient's finger, ensure that any nail vanish has been removed. This improves the connection.

If a diathermy plate is required you must ensure that it is in the correct position and in good contact with an area of dry skin. When the diathermy equipment is bipolar, as the one shown in Figure 2.8, there will *not be a plate* for the patient. This is because in this type the live and indifferent electrodes are incorporated within the diathermy forceps.

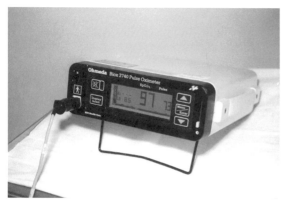

Figure 2.7 Pulse-oximeter. (Reproduced with permission from the Department of Medical Illustration, Ipswich Hospital NHS Trust, Ipswich, UK.)

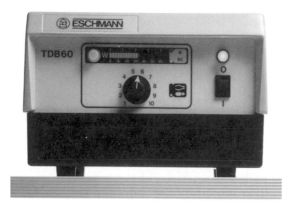

Figure 2.8 Eschmann diathermy. (Reproduced with permission from Eschmann Equipment, Lancing, UK.)

When you are arranging the diathermy equipment for use, you should also place the foot-operating pedal for the diathermy on the floor. This should be positioned at the foot end of the operating table where the podiatrist will be able to reach it when it is required without having to change position.

When an automatic tourniquet is being used, you should attach the lead from the ankle tourniquet to the machine (assuming that the cuff is in place on the ankle).

If an operating table patient foot rest is going to be required for the operation, this should also be placed in position before any of the surgical drapes are put in place.

> **TIP:** Foot rests are mainly employed when power equipment is used, often during bunion operations.

If a screen is going to be used then it should also be put into place at this time. Sometimes, however, instead of a full screen, only a frame or a Mayo table (Fig. 2.9) will be placed in front of the patient, and one of the surgical drapes will be attached to this to obscure the patient's view of their feet. In this case the frame or table will be put into place later (see p. 49 and Fig. 3.10).

Attending to the patient

First, you should think of the patient's dignity. In some theatres, for procedures other than nail avulsions, the patient will have taken off their outer clothing and be wearing only underwear and a theatre gown. If necessary, cover the patient with a draw sheet. Remember that the patient may also feel cold due to the air conditioning in the operating room.

Finally if there are any dressings on the patient's foot that have to be removed you must put on disposable gloves before removing these dressings. After doing this you should place the dressings, together with your gloves, into a disposal bag. As the operation has not yet started, the disposal bag can be removed from the theatre.

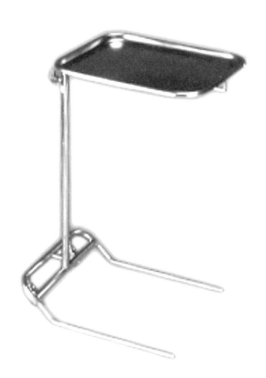

Figure 2.9   Mayo table. (Reproduced with permission from Timesco Surgical & Medical, London, UK.)

> **TIP:** Once the operation has started nothing must be taken out of the theatre.

IN THE THEATRE: THE OPERATION ABOUT TO START

When the surgical drapes have been placed over the patient by the surgical team, and the scrub assistant has the instrument trolley and instruments arranged to his or her satisfaction, you may be asked to provide any of the extras that will be required for the operation.

> **TIP:** Even if you know what is required you must wait for the scrub assistant to ask. Do not anticipate.

Instrument and suture packs provided by surgical suppliers are normally double wrapped. However, individual instruments that have been sterilized by the hospital sterilization depart-

ment may be in only a single transparent pack. If this is the case you must check that the single pack has not been punctured by the instrument. If you find that any of the packs have been damaged in any way then that pack must be discarded.

Irrespective of who supplied the instruments or dressings, each pack will generally have a visible autoclave tape, or colour changing area, on it. If the tape is broken or the colour has not changed then the contents must be considered unsterile and they must not be used.

> **TIP:** If the outer wrapper of an individual instrument pack was used as a dust cover this outer wrapper must be removed in the sterile store and not brought into the theatre.

When opening a sterile pack for the scrub assistant stand well back, holding the open end of the pack towards the person. Let the scrub assistant remove the contents, either with a gloved hand or with long-armed forceps (Fig. 2.10).

> **TIP:** Do not shoot or flick the contents of the pack on to the scrub assistant's trolley. Also, do not stand too near the trolley.

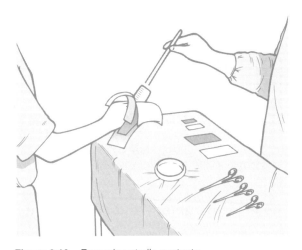

Figure 2.10   Removing sterile contents.

Pouring solutions

> **TIP:** When offering bottled solutions show the scrub assistant the label. You must both check the contents and the expiry date.

You should pour the liquid into the offered container from a height of at least 12 cm. Be careful, however, because the outside of the bottle you are holding is not sterile so you must not touch the offered container, nor the scrub assistant's gloves or gown.

An accepted method often used that allows the solution to remain sterile is to remove the cap and position the bottle over a kick basin, or sink. Then allow a small amount of the solution to run into the basin. Without interrupting the stream of liquid, the scrub assistant then places the sterile container into the stream until the container is filled to the desired level.

> **TIP:** Be careful not to place the bottle cap on the sterile table.

Drawing fluid from an ampoule

> **TIP:** Before opening the ampoule check that you are holding the correct drug. You must check this, as well as the expiry date, with both the podiatrist and scrub assistant.

First you should wipe the outside of the ampoule with an alcohol wipe. Then, using a piece of sterile gauze to protect your fingers, snap off the top of the ampoule. Now hold the ampoule in an inverted position (the fluid will not come out) to allow the scrub assistant to insert a transfer needle and withdraw the liquid. You must hold the ampoule in such a way that the scrub assistant's gloves do not touch it.

The first instrument and swab count

There are normally at least two instrument and swab counts during an operation, one before and one after the procedure. In addition, the scrub assistant may ask for further counts during the operation if there is a possibility that an instrument, suture or swab has been misplaced.

As the circulating assistant, one of your duties is to keep a record, both before and during the operation, of *all* the instruments, sutures and extras used during the operation. The purpose of this is to ensure that the number of items used is the same at the end of the operation as it was at the beginning and that no instrument or swab has been inadvertently left in the patient.

Instrument and swab counts are done by *both* the scrub assistant and the circulating assistant, and *one of you must be fully qualified*. Both of you must do the count together, and if either of you are uncertain about the total you must do a recount. Remember that all extra items used during the operation must be entered on to the count sheet.

> **TIP:** A very important point to remember is that no item may be removed from the operating theatre once the operation has started, and any item introduced after starting must be recorded on the count sheet.

Swabs should be counted in bundles of five, and you will find that the swabs in surgical instrument packs will normally have been tied in bundles of five by the sterilization department.

> **TIP:** The swabs you are using may have a black strip woven into them. This is known as a 'Raytec strip' and is detectable by X-ray.

The importance of the count sheet cannot be overemphasized as you will have to sign it. If a subsequent complication arises and a swab or instrument is found in the patient it is *you*, and not the podiatrist, who will have to explain the discrepancy at any inquiry.

> **TIP:** If an occasion ever arises in which a missing item fails to be found, you must fill in an incident form. For your own protection you are advised to make a photocopy of both the count

sheet and the incident form and keep them, in case there are future repercussions.

A word of warning: often in podiatric surgery, because of the operation site and the size of the incision, gauze squares are used in place of swabs. *These squares often come in packs of two.* If this is the case you should place the gauze pack covers to one side, and then use them to compare the number of gauze squares you have at the end of the operation with the total number of opened packs. *This must be done before dressing gauze squares are introduced into the sterile field to avoid the possibility of a mix-up between them.*

Setting up other theatre equipment

When the scrub assistant is ready you will be asked to help in preparing the scrub area by handing over any of the extra equipment that may be required during the procedure. By this time the podiatrist will have started to clean and prepare the surgical site. However, you must wait until you are asked before you move any equipment near the operating table.

The podiatrist finishes by painting the operation site with an antiseptic cleaning solution, often povidone–iodine (this solution is held in a sterile container, and applied with a swab that is normally held by sponge-holding forceps—Fig. 2.11).

After this has been completed, either the podiatrist or the scrub assistant will hand you the used container together with the sponge holder and swab. When taking the container and holder you

must take care not to touch the person's gloves or gown. Also, check with the scrub assistant whether the swab that was used for the solution application was from a surgical swab pack. If it was then that swab must then be counted in with the surgical swabs.

> **TIP:** In some operating theatres, racks (Fig. 2.12) are used to hold the discarded dirty surgical swabs, to simplify counting. Under no circumstances should a swab that was not from a surgical swab pack be placed on the rack.

When the podiatrist and the surgical assistant have draped the patient with the sterile drapes, the assistant will then hand you the trailing lead of the diathermy forceps. Taking care not to touch the 'greens', take the non-sterile end of the lead and attach it to the ports on the diathermy machine. Ask the podiatrist which settings are required, then adjust the controls on the diathermy machine to these settings. Then check that the foot-operating pedal is in the correct place for the podiatrist.

> **TIP:** It is a good idea to call out the settings on the diathermy so that both the podiatrist and the scrub assistant are aware of what you are doing.

If a Mayo table is to be used this can now be placed in position so that the scrub assistant can

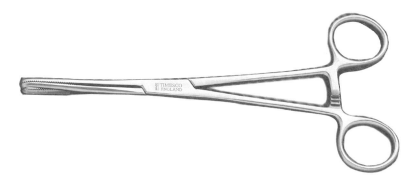

Figure 2.11   Rampley sponge-holding forceps. (Reproduced with permission from Timesco Surgical & Medical, London, UK.)

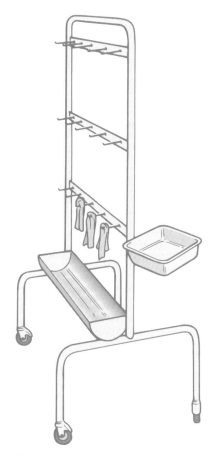

Figure 2.12   Swab rack.

cover it with a Mayo cover before laying out the instruments required for the operation.

When air-powered equipment is going to be used you will next be handed the air hose. However, before touching it check that you have been offered the correct end. Then plug the hose connector into the regulator on the air cylinder, but do *not* in any circumstances open the main cylinder valve to check the pressure or connection until you have been asked to do so by the scrub assistant or the person who is going to test the handpiece. After the pressure has been tested, you should close the main valve on the cylinder.

Once the operation has started, have a good look around to check whether everything is in place. Check also that the operating light is at the correct height. If you have to adjust the operating

light, be careful *not to touch* the sterile handle that is fitted in its centre (Fig. 2.13).

Maintaining the sterile field

As the circulating assistant you will not be wearing a sterile surgical gown, nor sterile gloves. So it is important that you do not inadvertently enter the sterile field and desterilize the drapes or equipment. Once something has been contaminated, it must not be used.

> **TIP:** A good practice is to imagine that there is an invisible barrier of about 30 cm around the sterile field and the surgical team, and you must not enter it. Give anything that is green a wide berth.

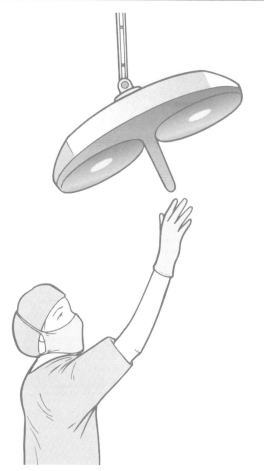

Figure 2.13   STOP! Only the scrubbed surgical team can touch this handle.

If you touch, or see anyone else who is not a member of the surgical team touch, a sterile surface, or if you see a member of the surgical team touch a non-sterile surface or object, *you must tell that person*. Do this even if it will result in the whole sterile field having to be changed, with the inevitable frustration and delay that this will cause, and especially if it is a special piece of apparatus that has become 'unsterile'.

> **TIP:** In some theatres 'the theatre greens' may actually be grey or even blue.

Generally speaking, consider anything green as sterile; this includes drapes on the patient and trolleys and the gowns worn by the scrub team. If in any doubt, don't touch; ask the scrub assistant first.

> **TIP:** Accidental desterilization is most likely to take place at the beginning of the operation, when trolleys are being positioned, and extra equipment and instruments are being placed or passed into or out of the sterile field.

You may find it helpful if you can try to visualize the invisible barrier described in the tip earlier when helping to move trolleys for the scrub assistant. Try to hold the trolley on the bare metal about 30 cm below the sterile drape. Take care that you do not come between the scrub assistant, or the podiatrist, and the trolley or operating table as you could inadvertently desterilize both of them. Also, never, never step backwards without looking.

> **TIP:** If you are watching the operation take care that you do not brush or allow your clothing to flap against the sterile drapes.

When the operation has been completed, don't be in a hurry to move or clear the scrub assistant's trolley. Wait until you are told to do so. Often the podiatrist, when finished, will state that the sterile field can be broken. That is normally the signal that the podiatrist is satisfied

that there are no complications, and that the equipment can be cleared away.

> **TIP:** Remember when you are clearing away equipment after the operation that, if a tourniquet has been used, it is also your duty to record the time the tourniquet was deflated.

Taking specimens from the scrub assistant

At times during the operation you may have to take a tissue specimen from the scrub assistant. It is important that you must use the correct container for the sample. Equally important, you must label the side of the container with the patient's name *before* the sample is placed in the container.

> **TIP:** Do not put the label on the lid, but always on the side of the jar. Lids can easily be taken off or put on to another jar by mistake.

Wearing gloves, you should hold the container well clear of but above the scrub assistant's trolley. This is to ensure that if the scrub assistant accidentally drops the sample it will not fall on to the floor but rather on to a sterile surface. From here it can hopefully be retrieved without too much damage to the specimen.

> **TIP:** At no time must you ever have more than one unlabelled container open. Also, never, never leave a specimen in a container if there is no label on the side of the container.

The label must show the patient's name, registration number, department or ward, name or type of specimen, date and time. The same information is entered on to the appropriate histology examination request card, which must be signed by the podiatrist. You may also find that your department keeps a theatre register of all samples that are sent to histology.

> **TIP:** Although some hospital histology departments issue specimen bottles with labels already attached, these labels are not universal and differ from hospital to hospital.

In podiatric surgery most tissue specimens are for histology, and will be placed in formol–saline. The correct level of the formol–saline should just cover the specimen. Microbiology specimens on the other hand are normally placed into a culture medium. *It is very important to remember that these specimens are a potential source of infection.* This applies not only to yourself but to others who may have to touch the container. Therefore, to reduce the risk of transferring any infection, as soon as you have labelled and sealed the container you should place it into a non-spill transporter bag.

> **TIP:** Specimens, including blood samples, must not be kept in a refrigerator that is used to store food or drink.

3

As a member of the scrub team

THE ROLE OF THE SCRUB ASSISTANT

The scrub assistant is often portrayed on film and TV as the nurse in the centre of the surgical team, controlling the action, remaining calm in any surgical situation and handing the correct instruments to the surgeon without having to be asked, and indeed there is a certain degree of truth in this image.

However, to achieve this degree of skill it should not be forgotten that the scrub assistant will most probably have spent a considerable time as a circulating assistant before becoming a scrub assistant. With the exception of specially trained chiropody assistants, the duties of the scrub assistant may also be carried out by podiatrists attached to the department or by student podiatric surgical pupils.

Even though you may have been working as a circulating assistant for some time, the change of role to that of scrub assistant (with different responsibilities) may at first seem a large jump. However, it is very unlikely that you will ever be asked to undertake the role of scrub assistant without having first assisted a trained scrub assistant or having a trained scrub assistant 'scrub in' with you. But if this should happen to you then just let the podiatrist know, so that the surgeon will be aware of your degree of experience.

Most podiatrists value a good scrub assistant, not only as an extra pair of hands but also because their expertise is invaluable during difficult operations. The experienced assistant should aim at giving the podiatrist a good clear, dry and clean operative site. Therefore the assistant must know how and when to mop, to remove clips, to follow continuous sutures without crossing the suture, to handle forceps and retractors, to cut sutures and to use the diathermy, all without obscuring the podiatrist's view.

In the early days remember: the better prepared you are, the less nervous you will be. Look at the surgical lists, notice which operations are the regular ones and, if possible, ask whether you can watch (from within the surgical field, and wearing a sterile gown and gloves) before you actually 'scrub in' as a member of the surgical team.

You should also take the time to read up on the various podiatric operations that are carried out in your department, and learn some of the anatomy of the foot (see Ch. 10). This will help you to make the transition go smoothly and be more interesting for you. *The wise surgical pupil will also consider time spent as a scrub assistant to be a valuable apprenticeship.*

SCRUBBING IN

Before you enter the operating room you must 'scrub up'—in other words you must wash and dry your hands and arms in a special way. This wash is carried out *before* putting on your gown and gloves, and your fingernails should be short and free from polish. (Damaged nail polish can harbour microorganisms.)

> **TIP:** The actual method used may differ slightly from hospital to hospital, so you are advised to follow your hospital's guidelines.

However, though the techniques may differ, if only in the duration of the actual wash, the basic principles remain the same: to remove dirt and bacteria from the hands and arms and to provide an antiseptic cover to the skin.

> **TIP:** If you wear spectacles you can stop them misting over if you place a small strip of sticking plaster over the upper edge of your mask (do this before you wash your hands).

The hand wash

1. Check that your hands and arms are free from cuts, skin rashes or eczema (eczematous dermatitis). If there is any break in the skin, then either *you should not scrub in* at all, or, if the wound is small, it must be covered (with a waterproof plaster) and you should double up on gloves.

> **TIP:** Whether or not you will be allowed to scrub in when you have a break in your skin will depend on the protocol of the facility that you are working in.

2. Remove all jewellery from hands or wrists (in some cases your wedding ring can stay on).
3. Turn the water on, but do not use your hands. You should be able to control the water flow by either a foot control or elbow taps. The water should be lukewarm and have a moderately forceful stream. Normally it is left running throughout the scrub.

The preparatory hand wash

4. Wash your hands and arms with an antiseptic soap or detergent designed for surgical scrubs for at least 30 seconds, holding your hands downwards.
5. Rinse thoroughly, then apply an antimicrobial agent, allowing it to lather on your arms. Leave this on.
6. Clean under your nails with a nail file or scraper under running water, then discard the nail file in the appropriate waste receptacle. *Do not allow your hands or arms to touch the sink or tap.*

The brush-stroke method

7. After rinsing your hands under the tap, take a brush with an impregnated antimicrobial

detergent. Wet it and begin the full scrub procedure, which involves scrubbing the hands and arms to above the elbow.

> **TIP:** Your hands, with the fingers pointing upwards, should be held higher than the elbows at all times, so that the water flows off at the elbows.

8. Holding the brush perpendicular to the nails of the left hand, scrub for 50 strokes in a backwards-and-forwards motion. Repeat this on the right hand.

9. Brush all four sides of each digit, using 10 strokes for each plane of each digit (i.e. 40 strokes per digit). The strokes should be curved to cover the space at the base of each finger.

> **TIP:** Should you drop your brush into the sink, leave it there and take another one.

10. Brush the front, back, inner and outer surfaces of the left hand (using 10 strokes for each surface). Repeat this for the right hand.

11. Brush the forearm from the wrist to about 5 cm (2″) above the elbow. Visualize your arm in three planes and brush each plane 10 strokes. Scrub one-third of each arm, alternating between the arms, and working backwards and forwards until you have completed the scrub to above the elbow.

12. Discard the brush.

13. Now thoroughly rinse your hands and arms under the tap, starting with the fingertips and proceeding over the arms and elbows. *Keep your hands at a higher level than your elbows.*

14. Stand for a moment to allow the excess water to drain off your elbows.

15. Proceed to the gowning area with your hands held at about eye level and well away from your body.

Some areas tend to be frequently missed during hand washing. These are shown in Figure 3.1.

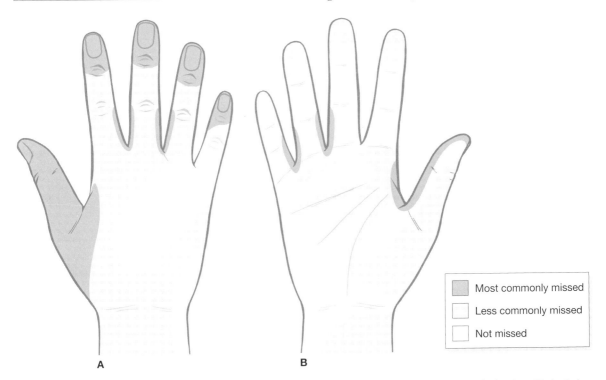

Most commonly missed

Less commonly missed

Not missed

A B

Figure 3.1 Areas frequently missed during hand washing. A: Back. B: Front. (Reproduced with permission from Taylor L J 1978 An evaluation of handwashing techniques—1. Nursing Times Jan 12, pp. 54–55.)

> **TIP:** In some hospitals the brush-stroke method is reserved for the first scrub of the day. Repeating this method throughout the day has the disadvantage of roughening the skin on the hands and arms, which brings organisms to the skin surface. If you need to scrub in for further operations, a less vigorous method known as the 'timed method' is often employed for subsequent scrubs. This uses only a sponge impregnated with an antimicrobial agent.
> Follow the policy for your hospital, as some podiatric units use only the timed method.

Timed method (5 minutes)

1. Wash your hands and arms with an antiseptic soap. There are a number of antiseptic agents in common use, such as povidone–iodine (e.g. Betadine®), chlorhexidine (e.g. Hibitane®), or hexachlorophane (e.g. Dermalex®, pHisoHex®). After this, rinse your hands and arms under running water.
2. Then, using an antimicrobial-impregnated sponge, wash your hands and arms to above the elbows for 2 minutes.
3. Rinse the lather off under running water.
4. Rescrub your hands, this time concentrating on the nails and fingers, for 1 minute (a sterile nail file and brush may be used at this stage).
5. Rinse your hands.
6. Now repeat the hand and arm wash for 2 minutes.
7. Finally rinse your hands and arms then, keeping your hands raised and away from your body, proceed to the gowning area.

Timed method (10 minutes)

As an alternative to the brush-stroke method as the 'first scrub' of the day, a number of surgical units employ the 10 minute timed scrub. This method is similar to that of the 5 minute scrub and is broken down into the following sequence.

(A) 1. Using an antimicrobial-impregnated sponge, wash your left hand for 1 minute.
    2. Then wash your left arm to above the elbow for $1\frac{1}{2}$ minutes.
    3. Rinse your left hand and arm.
(B) 1. Now wash your right hand for 1 minute.
    2. Then wash your right arm to above the elbow for $1\frac{1}{2}$ minutes.
    3. Rinse your right hand and arm.
(C) 1. Wash your left hand for 1 minute.
    2. Wash your left arm again, but this time to 5 cm (2″) above the elbow for 1 minute.
    3. Rinse your left arm and hand.
(D) 1. Wash your right hand for 1 minute.
    2. Wash your right arm to 5 cm (2″) above the elbow for 1 minute.
    3. Rinse your right arm and hand.
(E) Wash your left hand for 30 seconds. Then rinse.
(F) Wash your right hand for 30 seconds. Then rinse.

Finally, keeping your hands raised with fingers upwards, and away from your body, proceed to the gowning area.

Drying hands and arms after a surgical scrub

After the wash the circulating assistant will open a gown pack on to a table in such a way that you can pick up the sterile towel that should be lying on top of the gown (see Ch. 2, p 26–28). Most gown packs contain one or two towels.

> **TIP:** The gown is packed inside out, so that it can be laid on to a clean, but not necessarily sterile, surface with no danger of the outside of the gown being rendered unsterile.

Then, without dripping water onto the gown, as otherwise you will have to use another gown, dry your hands and arms as follows (Fig. 3.2):

1. Pick up the sterile towel. This towel is normally folded lengthwise. One end of the

towel is used to dry one hand (Fig. 3.2A). Use a blotting motion.

2. Rotate your arm and dry it from wrist to elbow (Fig. 3.2B).
3. Use the dried hand to hold the other end of the towel, and dry the other hand with this (Fig. 3.2C).
4. Then dry your second using the same blotting method as above (Fig. 3.2D).
5. Dry your elbows (Fig. 3.2E) and then discard the towel.

Alternatively, you can use two towels; here one towel is used for each hand and arm. In either event, once the towel has reached the elbow it is considered contaminated, and must not come into contact with a previously dried area of your hand or arm. Equally if the towel touches your clothes it is then considered contaminated and a new towel must be used.

GOWNING

There are two methods of gowning: with the assistance of the circulating assistant, as previously explained on pp 26–28, or with the assistance of a previously gowned person. (You could gown and glove yourself unassisted, but this is not recommended.)

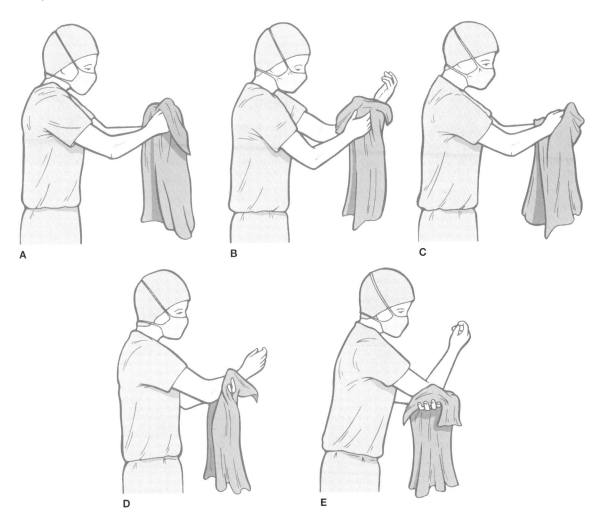

Figure 3.2 A–E: Drying hands and arms after a surgical scrub.

Assisted gowning by a previously gowned person (Fig. 3.3)

In this method the gowned person picks up a gown then, holding it by the neck ties, holds it at arm's length and allows it to unfold. The gown is held at shoulder height, with its sterile outside facing the gowned person and its inside facing you. You then put your arms into the arm holes on the gown, with your arms held upwards so that the gown stays in place. The person assisting can now fasten the back of the gown. If you are gloving using the closed-glove method, your hands should not emerge from the gown. Remember you cannot tie the waist ties until you have your gloves on.

GLOVING

Closed method

At first this appears to be a complicated way of putting on your gloves, but it is actually an easy, straightforward and practical way that allows you to put on your gloves with no danger of desterilizing them with your fingers.

The closed-glove method for a right-handed person (a left-handed person would start with the other hand) is as follows (Fig. 3.4).

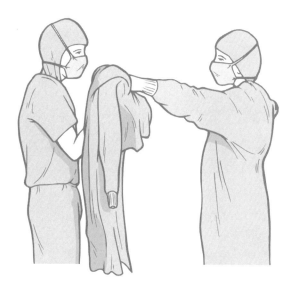

Figure 3.3 Gowning: assisted by a previously gowned person.

1. Your hands and fingers are covered with the gown. With your right hand, pick up the left glove and place it on your left wrist, glove thumb over hand thumb (palm uppermost) (Fig. 3.4A).

2. Pull the bottom of the glove over your hand until you can anchor it with your thumb, still in the gown (Fig. 3.4B). Now, with your right hand (covered by gown) pull the glove on to your left hand (Fig. 3.4C).

3. With your now-gloved left hand, pick up the right glove and place it on your right wrist (Fig. 3.4D). Hold the bottom edge of the glove with the fingers of your right hand (through the gown) (Fig. 3.4E) and, with your left hand, pull the glove over your right hand (Fig. 3.4F).

4. Adjust the fingers until the gloves fit correctly.

Open method

This method is often used when sterile gloves are required, possibly for redressing or suture removal, but when you are not wearing a sterile gown. Or it may be used after you have had to push your hands through the sleeves of the gown.

> **TIP:** You will notice that sterile gloves in the packs have the cuff folded over; this enables you to pick up the glove without touching the sterile outside of the glove.

The procedure is as follows (Fig. 3.5).

1. Pick up one glove by the cuff and slip your other hand into the glove (Fig. 3.5A).

2. Then, with the gloved hand, pick up the other glove by reaching *under* the folded cuff, *touching only the sterile surface of the glove with the previously gloved hand* (Fig. 3.5B).

3. You can now pull the glove on to the un-gloved hand (Fig. 3.5C) without your gloved hand touching the inside surface of the glove or your skin.

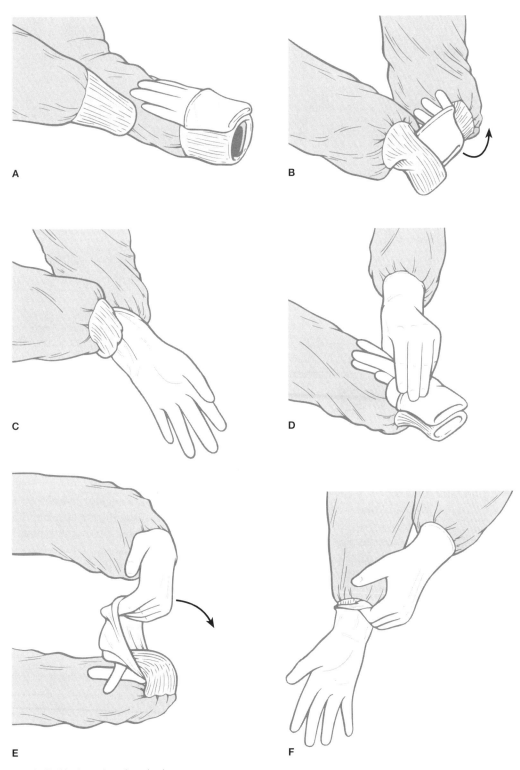

Figure 3.4   A–F: Gloving: closed method.

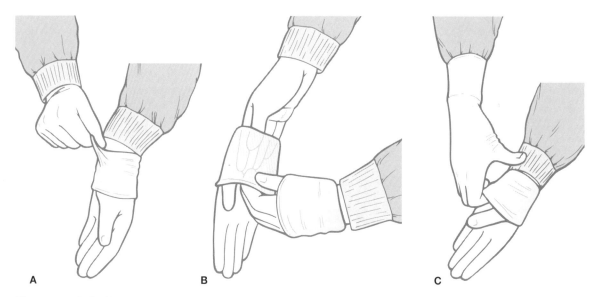

Figure 3.5 A–C: Gloving: open method.

Assisted method

Assisted gloving is normally used if you need to change gloves after accidental desterilization or glove damage when you are gowned up.

The procedure is as follows (Fig. 3.6).

1. A sterile member of the surgical team opens a sterile package and picks up a glove. Then, advising the recipient which hand to use, the person holding the glove holds the cuff of the glove and pulls the glove open, with the thumb of the glove towards the hand that is to be gloved (Fig. 3.6A).

2. Keeping the thumb close to the fingers (to avoid catching the glove), the recipient puts the hand into the glove using a forceful downward motion (Fig. 3.6B, C).

3. The procedure is repeated for the other hand, although this time the recipient can assist using the gloved hand (Fig. 3.6D).

> **TIP:** This can go wrong for the following reasons.
> 1. The recipient, instead of forcing the hand down, raises it as the glove starts to cover the hand. Note that it is the downward motion of the recipient's hand that puts the glove on, and not an upward motion by the person holding the glove.
>
> 2. The person holding the glove does not grasp the glove firmly enough to combat the force used by the recipient to push the hand into the tight-fitting glove.

POINTS ON STERILE TECHNIQUE

Having gowned and gloved there are a number of points that you should observe to remain sterile:

- gowns are considered sterile only on the sleeves between the elbow and hand and on the front of the gown from the waist upwards
- the back of the gown is considered to be unsterile (the exception is a gown with a back flap—see below)
- gowned staff must pass each other *back to back*
- keep your hands above waist level
- when gowned and gloved you can touch only sterile surfaces
- do not allow an unsterile person to reach over a sterile field
- do not allow an unsterile person to come between you and the operating table or the sterile instrument trolley
- anything that goes below the level of a sterile surface (including the operating table,

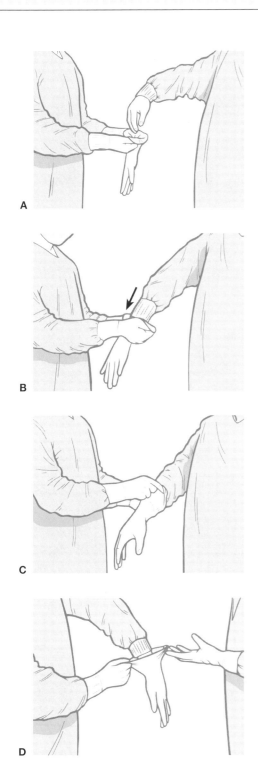

A

B

C

D

Figure 3.6   A–D: Gloving: assisted method.

instrument trolley and your waist) must be considered to be contaminated.

> **TIP:** If you are in any doubt about the sterility of any item of equipment or surface, consider it to be unsterile and either cover it or remove it from the sterile field.

Whereas some surgical gowns are open at the back, and therefore the back is unsterile, other types of gowns have a flap that allows you to cover your back. Wearing the latter type of gown will allow you to safely move between the trolley and the operating table, and turn your back on the trolley drapes without danger of desterilizing them.

> **TIP:** When you are wearing sterile surgical gloves keep your hands above waist level. If you don't know what to do with them, hold your hands together in front of your chest. In this way you are unlikely to touch an unsterile surface accidentally.

SETTING UP THE INSTRUMENT TROLLEY

When unwrapping the inner green sterile wrap of the instrument pack you will, unlike the circulating assistant, open the wrap first *towards* rather than *away from* yourself. In this way there will be a sterile green surface between you and the trolley, protecting your sterile gown as you lean across to open the rest of the wrap.

The sequence for opening the sterile instrument pack is as follows (Fig. 3.7).

1. The outer 'clean' cover has previously been opened by the circulating assistant (Fig. 3.7A; see also Fig. 2.6, p. 29).

2. Taking hold of the left edge of the green towel and taking care not to allow your gloves to touch the white paper cover, stretch out the left side of the green towel and allow its end to drape over the edge of the table (Fig. 3.7B).

3. Now do the same with the fold on the right side of the pack (Fig. 3.7C).

4. Now open the front fold towards yourself, allowing the fold to cover the complete front edge of the table (Fig. 3.7D).

5. Finally, open the rear fold so that the table top is completely covered with the green towel (Fig. 3.7E).

The overhang of the drapes should be about 30 to 50 cm all the way around the trolley. If this is not possible an extra green towel should be utilized.

At this stage you should consider the operation that is about to be undertaken, and the order in which the instruments will be used. You can lay out the instruments *in any order that you like*, but make sure that you can lay your hand on any instrument or piece of equipment without delay.

> **TIP:** Before you lay out your instruments, check with the podiatrist that there has been no change in the operation list, and whether any special instruments are going to be required.

When the basic instrument trolley is set up to your satisfaction, you are now ready for the circulating assistant to hand you the extras. Ideally you should use long-handled non-toothed forceps to take items that are handed to you, taking care to ensure that neither the forceps nor your hands touch a non-sterile surface (see Fig. 2.10, p. 31).

First instrument count

When you have all the extras that you think will be required (although it is always possible that the podiatrist will ask for something different) you should carry out your first count. *If you are a student or are untrained you must do this count with a trained member of staff.*

> **TIP:** Instrument packs and packs for saws, K-wire drivers, etc. should each contain a contents list within the pack. This list will have been made out by the hospital sterilization department when the items were packed. Check the items in the pack against the list. If it is correct the circulating assistant should sign it; if incorrect this must be mentioned and the fact entered on to the theatre log sheet.

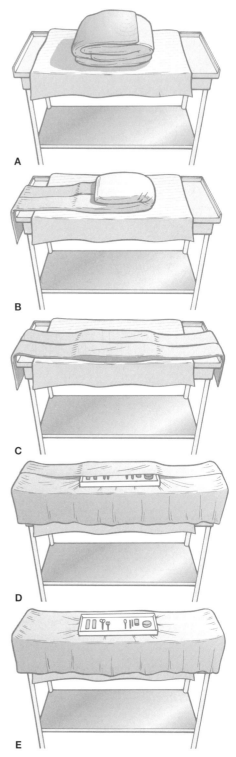

A

B

C

D

E

Figure 3.7 A–E: Opening an instrument pack.

When you have ensured that everything on the check list is present, you can ask the circulating assistant to add all of the extras to the list. Remember, if you are counting swabs in bundles of five, discard any bundles that have four or six swabs in them as they may confuse your count.

When sutures are used you may also consider keeping on one side of your trolley the sterile foil suture packets as an extra check on the number used.

Equally, the circulating assistant can keep the scalpel blade packets, and the outer pack covers of the prepacked gauze swabs if extra swabs are required. This is especially important when packs have less than five in them. Finally, remember that it is *you* and not the podiatrist carrying out the operation who is legally responsible for the count.

> **TIP:** If the circulating assistant opens scalpel blade packets in such a way as to allow the sterile blades to fall on to the instrument trolley, they should be dropped on to its right-hand corner.

PREPARATION OF THE PATIENT

When the trolleys are ready and the patient has been safely installed on the table, the podiatrist will ask for the skin preparation and cleaning lotion and sponge holders.

> **TIP:** Check that the proposed operation site corresponds to that entered on the consent form.

If you are asked to apply the lotion, then take care whilst doing this to avoid allowing your gloves or gown to touch either the operating table or the patient (neither of which is sterile). Ask the circulating assistant to lift the patient's foot that is going to be operated on. Then place a waterproof sterile towel over the table end and under the elevated foot, *and over the foot that is not going to be operated on.*

The circulating assistant then lowers the patient's foot on to the towel. (This towel can no longer be considered sterile.) You now apply the disinfectant lotion, which is often povidone–iodine, starting at the proposed incision site and working outwards from there, without going back on yourself. The foot should be 'painted' up to the edge of the ankle tourniquet if one is used. Such a large area is necessary even if only one toe is being operated on, so that adjustments can be made to the drapes without the podiatrist touching unprepared skin.

> **TIP:** Take care that you do not wash off any operation site indicator that is marked on the foot. This is especially important when the operation is for a soft tissue procedure, for instance an operation to excise an interdigital neuroma.

Draping the patient

Considerations you should observe when draping the patient include the following:

- do not place drapes on wet skin
- do not be in a hurry to apply the drapes; apply the proper technique for the operation that is going to be performed
- handle the drapes as little as possible
- drapes should be carried folded to the operating table, taking care not to touch any non-sterile surface
- drape the area around the incision first; draping should always be done from a sterile area to an non-sterile area.

> **TIP:** Sterile drapes are often referred to as green towels, or GTs, even though they may actually be another colour.

You are now ready to place the sterile drapes around the patient. Ask the circulating assistant to lift the patient's foot once more. The circulating assistant should do this taking care not to touch the painted skin, otherwise it will have to be repainted. A second circulating assistant can then remove the waterproof towel that was used during the application of the paint.

> **TIP:** Remember that no member of the 'scrubbed' surgical team can touch this towel as it is now considered unsterile.

The circulating assistant continues to hold the foot off of the table whilst the waterproof towel is replaced with a fresh sterile one before you continue to drape the foot. The following method is often employed for this. It is explained here in detail *as one example* of draping the patient.

> **TIP:** Different departments/hospitals or podiatrists may use other methods.

With the foot to be operated on still elevated and held by the circulating assistant and the 'dirty' waterproof towel having been removed, you, as the scrub assistant, should take hold of one end of a fresh waterproof sterile towel and hold the other end out to the podiatrist. Then together you open and place this fresh towel, as before, under the foot that is to be operated on, but over

the patient's other foot, which is still resting on the table. Next take a large green towel and give one end of this to the podiatrist, then open it out and together fold the towel so that one-third of the towel folds back on itself (Fig. 3.8).

This double layer is then placed under the foot to be operated on, with its open end towards the foot end of the table—in other words towards yourself, but you should also lay this towel over the foot that is not going to be operated on. This will prevent that foot from coming into direct contact with the other foot or any sterile surface or equipment. The foot that is to be operated on is then lowered on to the drape. Finally, you and the podiatrist should take and unfold a second large green towel. Holding it above the patient's leg and foot, but not touching the foot, both of you now position the towel so that it not only covers the patient's leg and foot but also extends approximately 50 cm beyond the foot end of the operating table. When the towel is in position allow it to drop and drape over the complete foot and end of the table (Fig. 3.9). (The table end is protected by the first sterile drape.)

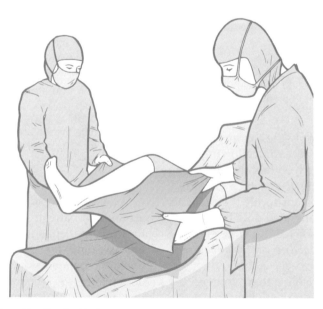

Figure 3.8 Draping the foot: making the double layer.

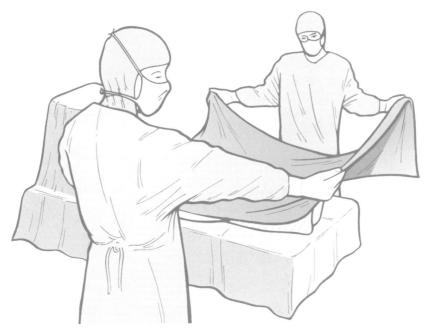

Figure 3.9   Draping the foot: top drape.

> **TIP:** It is a good idea to hold the green towel over the area to be covered and allow it to drape over the area by letting it go. This allows gravity to place it in position, rather than you bending and allowing your hands to go below the level of the operating table, so there is less chance of your accidentally touching either the patient or the operating table.

A further drape can be placed over the patient so that if required this can form a screen for the patient (Fig. 3.10).

You or the podiatrist can now roll the edge of the top drape so that it is held against the edge of the upper folded portion of the lower drape. These rolled edges are then held together with four towel clips. A clip is placed on either side of the foot to hold the drape close to the skin (Fig. 3.11).

A further two clips are used to hold the drapes together approximately 30 cm from each side of the foot. This will allow the podiatrist to elevate the foot to be operated on with no danger of the sterile glove touching any part of the patient's other foot or leg.

> **TIP:** Once the towel clip has penetrated the towel, that clip cannot be removed and reused, as the portion of the clip that has penetrated the towel is now considered to be unsterile.

When the foot is elevated the lower fold of the folded towel will stay in place covering the end of the operating table and the patient's other foot.

This procedure may at first appear to be confusing or difficult to do without getting your hands contaminated, but don't worry—with a little practice you will soon be proficient.

> **TIP:** A fifth towel clip may be used as an anchor for the diathermy lead or the hose for an air-driven saw (Fig. 3.12).

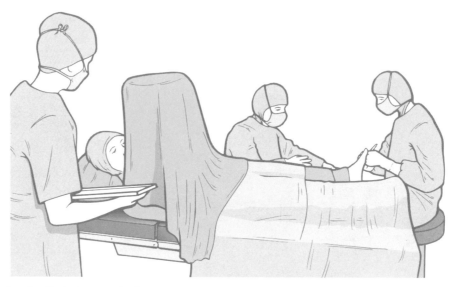

Figure 3.10 Draping the foot: screen in place.

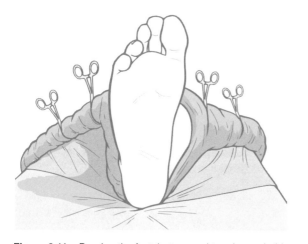

Figure 3.11 Draping the foot: bottom and top drapes held together with towel clips.

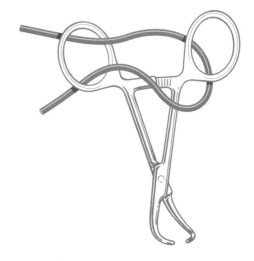

Figure 3.12 Method of attaching a lead to a towel clip.

Using waterproof paper drapes

Some hospitals have replaced material (cloth) green towels with paper waterproof sterile drapes; these may be green, grey or light blue in colour. If these are used there are some points that you should consider when the operation is being undertaken with the patient under a local anaesthetic.

When cloth green towels are used, any fluid including blood will be absorbed by the towel and show as a dark stain. It is therefore not seen by the patient as an obvious bloodstain. However, a waterproof paper towel is non-absorbent, and will allow blood or other fluids to pool in the folds of the towel. If the blood is mixed with the spill from, for example, a surgical flush this could possibly be seen by the patient as an alarming blood loss.

Another problem is that when you undrape these non-absorbent towels from the patient you may find that fluid or blood that has formed a pool in the folds of the towel then runs off the drape and over your shoe.

> **TIP:** When using waterproof paper towels, have an absorbent swab or towel ready to hold under the foot to absorb any spillage of blood or excess flush.

Generally speaking, however, a tourniquet is frequently used during podiatric operations so little bleeding occurs. Although most podiatric operations can be carried out *without* the use of a tourniquet, even during bunion procedures if carried out competently, using one ensures there will be little blood loss.

TESTING OF THE EQUIPMENT

After the patient is draped and the instruments have been laid out, the podiatrist will test the power saw or other power equipment before commencing the operation.

> **TIP:** Most saws must have the blade attached before testing. You should fit the blade to the saw with the latter held over a sterile cover, so that if you accidentally drop the blade it will fall on to the sterile surface with no danger of becoming desterilized.

You must make sure that the safety catch is on, or that the instrument is disconnected from its power source, *before attaching the blade*. After the saw, or other instrument, has been tested, the complete handpiece may be removed from the hose and placed on the trolley ready for use with the blade in position.

If a K-wire driver or a drill is to be used, this must also be tested prior to starting the operation. The podiatrist may also ask you to load the K wire.

The podiatrist will test the diathermy forceps. Quivers are sometimes used, and after testing the podiatrist will place the diathermy forceps into the quiver for easy access and to avoid the danger of the forceps falling off the table.

> **TIP:** When stools are used by the surgical team remember that, even if the stool is covered by a sterile drape, you must not allow any part of your gown above your waist or your gloves to touch this drape as it is considered to be unsterile. Even though the stool is considered clean, if it has to be repositioned the circulating assistant must still hold it below the level of the drape.

4

Assisting during the operation

THE SURGICAL ASSISTANT

It is quite possible when you are experienced as a scrub assistant or a surgical student you may be asked to act as the podiatrist's surgical assistant during the operation, as well as simultaneously carrying out the duties of the scrub assistant. This in some ways will depend on your training and qualifications as well as local rules and regulations. You are of course perfectly entitled to refuse to act as a surgical assistant if you have not been specifically trained in this role, or if you do not feel confident to do so.

USING AN ANKLE TOURNIQUET

It is a fairly common practice in podiatric surgery to use an ankle tourniquet for procedures other than nail surgery, when a Penrose tourniquet would be used (Fig. 4.1).

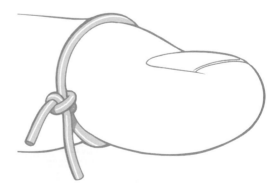

Figure 4.1 Penrose tourniquet.

If an ankle tourniquet is going to be used the foot will have to be exsanguinated and you will be asked to elevate the foot (now you will see the advantage of that double bottom wrap) whilst the podiatrist wraps an Esmarch bandage (a large rubber bandage approximately 6 cm wide and a metre in length) around the foot, starting over the toes and working up towards the ankle (Fig. 4.2).

The podiatrist will then ask the circulating assistant to inflate the tourniquet to the required pressure. This pressure is usually 70–120 mmHg above the patient's systolic blood pressure. Only after the tourniquet is inflated and the circulating assistant informs you that the pressure is stable can the patient's foot be lowered and the Esmarch bandage removed.

> **TIP:** The circulating assistant must record the pressure and the time that the tourniquet was inflated. The circulating assistant should also remind the podiatrist after each 20 minutes of tourniquet time have passed during the operation.

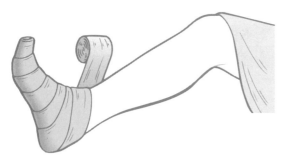

Figure 4.2   Esmarch bandage.

You are now ready to start.

PASSING INSTRUMENTS

Hand the podiatrist a toothed dissecting forceps, which are sometimes referred to as 'pick-ups' (Fig. 4.3).

> **TIP:** Forceps with serrated jaws must not be used as skin-holding retractors, because the serrated jaws will crush the skin.

The podiatrist will use the forceps to confirm that the patient cannot feel any sharpness (the podiatrist may also have tested for sensitivity before the tourniquet was inflated). When the podiatrist is satisfied you should pass the scalpel.

> **TIP:** In the unlikely event that the patient still feels pain and a further amount of anaesthetic is required, the circulating assistant should advise the podiatrist of the total amount that has previously been administered as entered on the preoperative check-sheet. This will ensure that the maximum safe dose is not exceeded.

Instruments should be passed in such a way that they can be used without the podiatrist having to look up (this takes practice). This is achieved by pressing the instrument firmly into the podiatrist's palm in such a way that the recipient will not drop it, nor be cut by the instrument. If either the surgeon's or your glove is damaged by the instrument then that instrument must be discarded immediately and the glove changed.

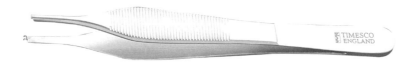

Figure 4.3   Toothed (Adson) dissecting forceps. (Reproduced with permission from Timesco Surgical & Medical, London, UK.)

When passing artery forceps, tissue scissors, or in fact any instrument with a scissor type of handle, you should hold the instrument close to the joint keeping the blades together. If the instrument is curved, pass it with the curve facing inwards (i.e. towards the podiatrist's other hand).

Retractors are held at the midpoint and passed in such a way that the handle goes into the podiatrist's hand with the blade pointing down towards the wound.

Toothed dissecting forceps are passed with the points downwards and held on the lower half, keeping the points closed. In this way the podiatrist can take hold of them at the top near the joint and ready for use.

Needle holders are passed in a similar manner to that of other scissor-type instruments.

The needle should be mounted with the curve of the needle at right angles to the needle holder and so that the needle holder grasps the needle just slightly to one side of the half-way point of the curve *on the same side as the thread*, with the point of the needle facing inwards (i.e. towards the podiatrist's other hand) (Fig. 4.5) (see also Ch. 7, p. 84 for proper loading of needles).

As you pass the needle holder you should hold the end of the thread to prevent it becoming desterilized (i.e. by its end dropping below the level of the operating table) or tangled.

ASSISTING AT SURGERY

In order to describe the role of the surgical/scrub assistant more easily, let us imagine that you are assisting at the reduction of a simple metatarsal

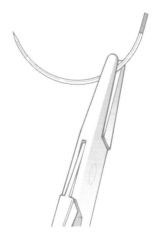

Figure 4.5 The suture needle is held slightly to one side of the halfway point of the curve.

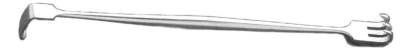

Figure 4.4 Kilner retractor. (Reproduced with permission from Timesco Surgical & Medical, London, UK.)

medial exostosis (Fig. 4.6). This procedure is sometimes called a Silver's bunionectomy.

Before the first incision is made you should have attached blades to at least two scalpel handles (often in podiatric surgery a no. 15 blade is used in conjunction with a no. 3 handle).

Mounting blades

The uninitiated tend to shudder when they watch podiatrists changing blades as they tend to use their fingers. This is a habit that most have picked up during their time in podiatry school and it is something that is unlikely to change.

You, on the other hand, should use a needle holder or forceps to change the blade (Fig. 4.7). To do this, grip the blade near the top end of its cut-out hole with the forceps. Then slide the

raised groove on the end of the handle into the cut-out on the blade (Fig. 4.8). Press the two together; the blade should now be firmly in position.

Before the first incision is made you may also have attached a blade to the surgical saw, and tested the power supply. Experience will tell you which blade you are going to need, but even so be prepared for the podiatrist to ask for a different blade size.

TIP: It may also be advisable to load three suture holders: one with a 2/0 dissolvable suture, another with a 3/0 dissolvable suture and a third with a 3/0 non-dissolvable suture.

The first incision

Podiatry surgical students, although already used to handling scalpels in their regular work,

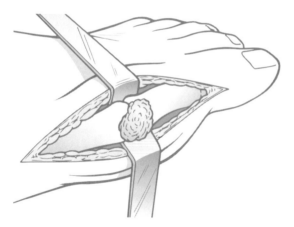

Figure 4.6   Metatarsal medial exostosis, retractors in place.

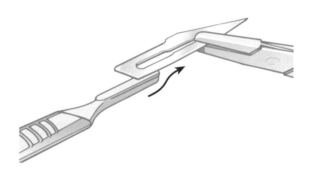

Figure 4.8   Mounting the blade.

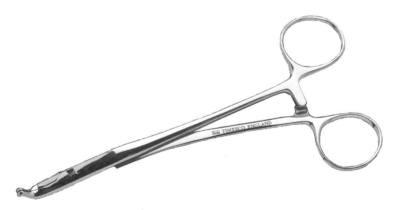

Figure 4.7   Scalpel blade applier and remover. (Reproduced with permission from Timesco Surgical & Medical, London, UK.)

generally do not hold the scalpel in a way that is appropriate to surgery. If the scalpel is held in a 'chiropody manner' it will produce an oblique cut as opposed to the sharp perpendicular incision that is required in surgery.

In surgery the scalpel is principally held in one of two ways: the knife grip or pen grip. The knife grip (Fig. 4.9) is used for cutting through thick tissue such as a capsule. Here the scalpel is held like a knife with the thumb against the middle and ring finger, and the index finger on the top of the scalpel handle to provide pressure and control.

The pen grip (Fig. 4.10) is probably the more commonly used grip in podiatric surgery, as it allows for smaller and more complicated controlled incisions. The handle is held like a pen. The amount of pressure applied when making the incision should be just enough to divide the epidermis and dermis down to the underlying fat. The incision should be done in one firm stroke, as repeated light strokes will produce an irregular incision.

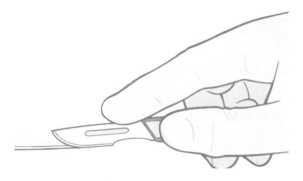

Figure 4.9 Knife grip.

When you have handed over the scalpel the podiatrist will make the first incision, medial to the extensor hallucis longus and over the exostosis. This first incision will often be a curvilinear incision of approximately 6 to 9 cm in length. After the skin incision has been made, you should take the first scalpel from the podiatrist and hand over a new one. The reason for this is that the skin may well have blunted the scalpel edge, and a new blade will be less likely to carry skin debris into the wound.

> **TIP:** You should have a sterile swab at hand for immediate use.

The podiatrist will now hold the wound open with toothed dissecting forceps, in a grip known as a 'pincer grip' (Fig. 4.11), to divide the superficial fat and expose the tissue over the capsule.

At this stage you may be asked to place a retractor over the now-exposed extensor tendon, and gently pull it away from the incision. The podiatrist will wish to protect the tendon as well as the dorsal digital nerve of the great toe, which runs parallel to the tendon, and this retraction will give the surgeon a clear view when making the next incision down to the level of the capsule.

If you see that a blood vessel is about to be cut you should have the diathermy forceps ready in your hand, as the podiatrist may wish to coagulate the bleeding points. If the podiatrist asks for a 'dab', dab the swab on to the bleeding point. Do *not* wipe it (this would

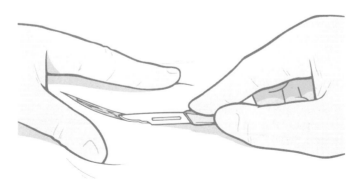

Figure 4.10 Pen grip.

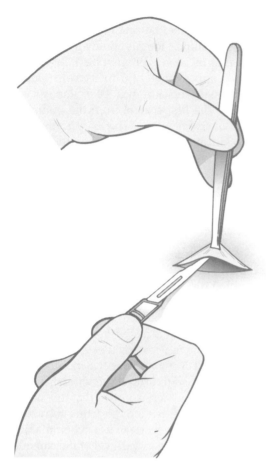

Figure 4.11   Toothed dissecting forceps held in the pincer grip.

dislodge any clot that may have formed). Often a straight in-and-out movement is all that is required. If the podiatrist asks for a 'wet dab', you should slightly dampen the swab with sterile saline or sterile water before dabbing. Then discard the swab into the swab bin and *not* on to your sterile trolley.

Controlling a cut blood vessel

If a blood vessel is cut, you may have to hand the podiatrist some artery forceps (called a haemostat) or a tie—which is a thin thread, size 3/0 or 4/0, without needles and made of a dissolvable material, possibly polyglycolic acid (see Ch. 7, p. 82). The procedure is as follows.

Ligation of a blood vessel

If a blood vessel is severed you should first hand the podiatrist a haemostat; this is used to clamp the tip of the vessel. The podiatrist will then pass the forceps handle back to you. You should hold the forceps vertically whilst the surgeon passes a length of suture material behind the forceps and down to the tip of the forceps (Fig. 4.12). Now depress the forceps handles, which raises the end of the blood vessel. The suture can now be passed under the points of the forceps and around the vessel, and the first knot tied. On an instruction from the podiatrist gently release the forceps, but maintain a soft grip on the vessel as the knot is completed. Remove the forceps only when asked.

> **TIP:** A blood vessel can also be tied off with a regular dissolvable suture such as a 3/0 Dexon®. You may find it convenient to have a needle holder loaded with a suture but without a needle, ready for immediate use. A needle holder will not always be required, however, as hand tying is often the preferred method.

Planned division of a blood vessel

In certain circumstances the surgeon may wish to cut through a large blood vessel (normally a

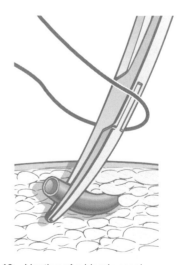

Figure 4.12   Ligation of a blood vessel.

vein). In this case you may be asked to use a haemostat as a retractor. You or the podiatrist will then place a haemostat with the tips on either side of the blood vessel that is to be cut. As you open the jaws of the forceps the tissue on either side of the vessel will be forced apart, exposing the vessel (Fig. 4.13A). Whilst you continue to hold the forceps in place, a second forceps is placed around the vessel and closed to occlude the vessel. The vessel is then ligated on either side of the forceps, and then cut between the ligatures (Fig. 4.13B).

Freeing the surrounding tissue

Before opening the joint capsule the podiatrist may wish to free the surrounding tissues. In this situation either the scalpel will be used or you will be asked for a pair of round-tipped curved Metzenbaum or Mayo scissors (Fig. 4.14). The closed blades of the scissors are inserted between the capsule and superficial tissues and the blades are then opened to tease the tissue off the capsule.

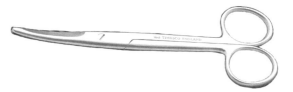

Figure 4.14 Mayo scissors, curved round point. (Reproduced with permission from Timesco Surgical & Medical, London, UK.)

When sufficient tissue has been released you may have to insert another retractor into the wound to improve the podiatrist's view whilst slicing through the capsule.

Keeping the instrument trolley tidy

Remember that even though you are assisting during the operation at all times you should try to keep your instrument trolley tidy. Avoid covering it with discarded swabs or overlapping instruments. However, always ask the podiatrist to hand back used instruments. Discarded blades and needles should be kept to one side, normally the left side of the instrument table in a gallipot, although in some departments a 'sticky mat' is used in place of this for the needles and blades. Either method will allow you to stop the used blades from becoming mixed up with the sterile blades.

> **TIP:** Something that you should be aware of, and should not allow, is the unacceptable habit of some podiatrists of allowing a number of instruments and dirty swabs to accumulate in a pile between the patient's legs. This is not only bad practice, but is also positively dangerous to the surgical staff as well as the patient.

Passing the saw

When the podiatrist has made the incision through the capsule and released it from the underlying bone this exposes the exostosis. After examining the exostosis the podiatrist will then decide which is the best blade to use on the saw. If a different blade is required and not the one you have already attached, load the saw with the

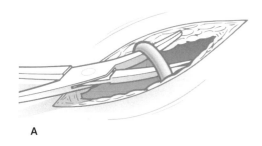

A

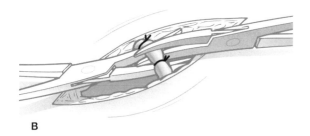

B

Figure 4.13 A, B: Planned division of a blood vessel.

new blade whilst holding the handpiece over your trolley. Then attach the handpiece to the hose. If the handpiece is already attached to the hose, you should ensure that the safety catch is on. It is *safer still to remove the hose before attaching the blade* and to ask the circulating assistant to open the air valve on the air bottle *only when you are ready and with the new blade in place.*

> **TIP:** When power tools are being used you should, for your own protection, wear a mask with a visor or goggles as there is the danger of blood, bone or tissue particles being thrown into the air.

When you are asked, pass the saw to the podiatrist. You may once again at this point have to use a retractor to assist in holding the wound open.

Using retractors

Retractors, as their name implies, are used to retract tissue back from the edge of the wound. They come in all shapes and sizes. Some have small hooks and are useful for delicate tissue handling; you may use these when assisting during a digital arthroplasty. Some are flat and others have curved ends. Irrespective of the shape, however, the same principle applies: you should hold the retractor *so that the tissue is not crushed*.

In this instance you may be asked to place a flat-bladed retractor under the head of the metatarsal, between the bone and the soft tissue (Fig. 4.15). In this position, as well as giving good exposure to the exostosis, the retractor will protect the underlying soft tissue, in the event that the saw blade inadvertently penetrates beyond the bone.

After the bone has been cut, take the bone fragment and place it into a gallipot. *Do not discard it with the dirty swabs.* If the metatarsal head is found to contain small sinuses (holes) the podia-

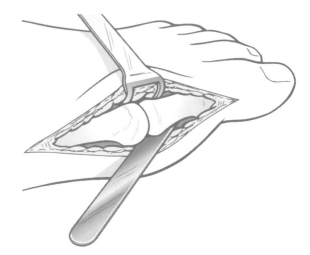

Figure 4.15 Flat-bladed metatarsal retractor in place.

trist may wish to break the bone fragment into smaller particles to pack into these holes.

After cutting the bone the podiatrist may ask for a bone rasp; this is a form of file and is shown in Figure 4.16.

At certain stages during the operation you may find that you are standing around with nothing more to do than to hold a swab. This is a good time to observe what the podiatrist is doing so that you can learn to anticipate what is needed. This will certainly help you at your next operation.

> **TIP:** Something to remember when you are watching is not to become so engrossed that you lean on the patient's legs.

You may also wish to take this time to remove or change the used scalpel blades and generally tidy up your trolley.

Removing blades

You may find this to be more difficult than mounting the blades. This time you should hold the handle so that the sharp edge of the blade is

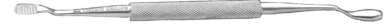

Figure 4.16 Bell (bone) rasp. (Reproduced with permission from Timesco Surgical & Medical, London, UK.)

pointing away from you and downwards. In other words, the blade should be lower than the handle (Fig. 4.17). Then, with either the needle holder or forceps, grip the blade just below the raised area on the handle. Now gently lift the end of the base of the blade over the raised area, and the blade should come off. Take care that no one is in front of you as the blade can suddenly spring off.

When the podiatrist has finished with the saw, disconnect the hose and place the handpiece on the trolley. You can keep the blade in place. The hose should be kept in place on the operating table (possibly held by a towel clip) until the operation is finished.

Before closing the wound the podiatrist will copiously flush the site with a surgical flush (possibly 0.02% gentamicin in saline). You should now hand the podiatrist a syringe which you have previously loaded with the flush.

Closing the wound

After flushing the wound the podiatrist will be ready to close it. At this point you will have to pass the needle with the 2/0 Vicryl® as this is the thicker thread and will be used for closing the joint capsule. At the same time you may have to continue holding the wound open with a retractor.

> **TIP:** In most operations the thicker thread is the one used first.

After each suture either you or the podiatrist will have to cut the suture. Internal sutures are cut a fraction above the knot.

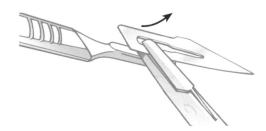

Figure 4.17 Removing blades.

> **TIP:** To cut sutures without cutting the knot you should pass the blades down the thread whilst holding them parallel to the tissue until you are just above the knot; then turn the blade edges upwards at about 45° to the thread and cut the suture.

If, because of anatomical structures, the internal suture is located in a place where the podiatrist finds it difficult to fasten the suture or tie the knot, you must take special care not to cut through the knot, or to be so close to the knot that there is a possibility that movement of the tissues may cause the thread to slide and untie the knot. In this situation the thread should be cut at least 4 mm from the knot.

In some situations, for instance when closing a deep wound or if it is difficult to fasten the last few sutures with a needle holder, the podiatrist may decide to hand tie all or some of the sutures. In this case a procedure called 'cut and clip' (Fig. 4.18)

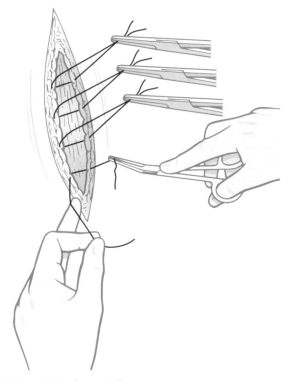

Figure 4.18 Cut and clip.

may be used. In this, the first suture is put in place and pulled through until there are equal lengths, going in and coming out. The podiatrist will then ask for artery forceps. You should place the artery forceps so as to hold both lengths of thread, and towards the end of the shorter length of thread. Then cut the longer thread, which has the needle attached; this can then be used for the next suture. After cutting the thread lay the forceps on the side of the wound. Take care to avoid allowing the weight of the forceps to pull on the thread. The podiatrist will work up the length of the incision, asking for new forceps for each thread. As you gain experience you will come to know in which operations this technique will be employed so you will have the required number of forceps available.

First closing count

Toward the end of the operation you should check your trolley and prepare for your first closing count. Don't be rushed by the podiatrist, it is very unlikely that the procedure cannot be stopped for a moment. You must count all the instruments, needles and swabs. Count out loud together with the circulating assistant. When you are sure that everything is present, tell the podiatrist. The podiatrist *must acknowledge this* before closing the wound.

> **TIP:** Don't forget to include the instruments, sutures or swabs that the podiatrist is using whilst you are carrying out your count.

Missing instruments

If something is found to be missing the podiatrist will stop closing whilst a search for it takes place. You must search for the missing item in every conceivable place: on the floor, stuck to the sole of someone's shoe, on the table, under the table, between the drapes, under containers, and even in the podiatrist's surgical boot.

If it is not found then no one should leave the theatre, and either you or the circulating assistant will now have to search through all of the surgical rubbish, including the swabs. The circulating

assistant should lay a waterproof paper sheet on the floor before tipping the swabs out. Wearing gloves, and preferably using forceps, the assistant should lay the swabs out, again in bundles of five. Be very careful if you are looking for a needle as it could easily have become imbedded into the swab. You must go through *everything* until the item is found. If it is still not found the podiatrist must be informed, and an incident report filled in. This should be signed by everyone in the surgical team including the circulating assistant.

Even whilst you are counting you must continue to pass the required instruments or sutures to the podiatrist. You may find this easier if you have loaded the needle holders and laid them out in the order of use before starting your count.

Assuming that all is well with your count, the next suture required will possibly be a 3/0 Dexon® dissolvable type. The podiatrist will use this to close the successive layers of the wound. You may also have to load a 4/0 Dexon® if a continuous subcuticular closure is going to be carried out, or a 3/0 Ethilon® if external sutures are going to be used. (Sutures are explained in Ch. 7 in more detail.)

> **TIP:** When cutting the external sutures, cut the thread at least half a centimetre from the knot. Remember that you may be the person who has to remove them, and if the ends are cut too close to the knot they may become imbedded in the scab. This makes them difficult to locate. (It is also painful for the patient.)

If a subcuticular closure is chosen you may also need Steristrips®; these give added support to the skin edges. (Further details of adhesive skin closures are given in Ch. 7, p 83–84.)

> **TIP:** Spray a small amount of Opsite® spray on to a swab, then gently rub the swab on either side of the incision site (Fig. 4.19A) before attaching the Steristrips® (Fig. 4.19B)—the Opsite® deposit will help the Steristrips® to adhere to the skin.

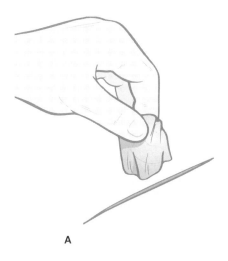

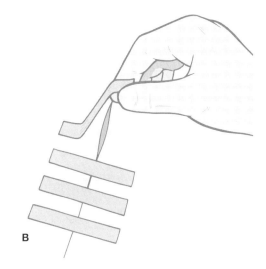

Figure 4.19   A: Opsite® and B: Steristrip® application.

By this stage you should have instructed the circulating assistant to prepare, but not as yet to hand you, the outer dressings.

Before placing the sterile dressing on the foot the podiatrist will normally clean the preoperative cleaning substance off the patient's foot. (In some instances the preoperative 'paint' may become an irritant to the patient if it is left on the skin for any length of time.) You should therefore have ready a swab soaked in sterile water or saline, and also a fresh dry one, to dry the foot. If some form of 'non-stick' dressing is requested, pass this to the podiatrist *before* passing the first wound dressing.

> **TIP:** Some podiatrists deflate the tourniquet before applying the dressings. In this case have a swab handy just in case there is a haemorrhage.

When the wound is closed you may disconnect the diathermy equipment. However, do not be in a hurry to remove the drapes as the podiatrist may wish to check whether there is any marked postoperative bleeding after the tourniquet has been released. If all is well, the podiatrist may

then declare that the 'toes are pink' and that the sterile field can be broken. This is a sign that the outer dressing can now be placed over the sterile dressings on the foot.

When preparing to 'clear away' drapes or instruments, you must at no time allow your hands to touch any non-sterile surface, which includes the outer dressing, until the podiatrist has stated that the sterile field can be broken.

> **TIP:** If the outer dressing is a 34 Tubinette® the length required for the average foot is calculated as the width of your body plus the length of one arm.

POSTOPERATIVE PROCEDURE

Depending on local protocol you, or possibly the second circulating assistant, will take the patient to the postoperative recovery room. Ensure that all relevant paperwork, the X-rays and the completed count sheet go with the patient. If the patient is to be transferred to a ward then any instructions that the podiatrist may have should also accompany the patient. The surgical register must now be filled in; this is a *legal document* that records the operation, type of anaesthetic used, the patient's name and number and the members of surgical staff who were present. It is a fact of life that abbreviations are sometimes used when filling in the surgical report (see Appendix 1, p. 135); however, generally speaking, abbreviations should be avoided, as they could cause serious ambiguity.

Removing the contaminated garments

Removing the contaminated gown

Contaminated gowns and gloves will normally be removed before you leave the operating room. If your are right handed, the procedure for removing your gown will be as follows, and as illustrated in Figure 4.20. Left-handed persons will start with the other hand. You will still be wearing your gloves, which must not be removed until after you have removed the gown.

1. The circulating assistant releases the back ties of the gown.

2. With your left hand, reach over to your right shoulder and pull the gown down to release your right arm and hand (Fig. 4.20A). Take care not to allow the outside of the gown to touch your scrub suit.

3. With your right hand, grasp the left shoulder (Fig. 4.20B) and pull the gown down; while holding it away from your scrub suit release your left arm and hand. Then allow the top half to fold over the lower part of the gown, at all times keeping the inner part of the gown towards you (Fig. 4.20C). Finally, touching the inside of the gown only, dispose of the gown in an appropriate container.

Removing the contaminated gloves

The procedure is as follows (Fig. 4.21).

1. Allow the cuffs of the gloves to fall forward. Then with one hand place the finger between the cuff and the palm of the other hand (Fig. 4.21A). Now pull the glove over the hand without allow-

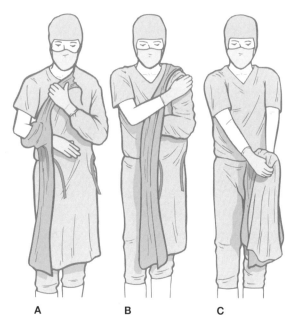

Figure 4.20 A–C: Removing a contaminated gown.

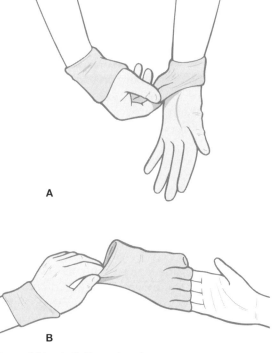

Figure 4.21 A–C: Removing gloves.

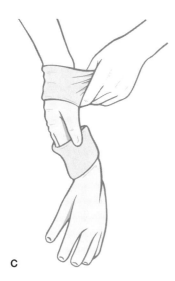

C

Figure 4.21

ing that hand to touch the outside of the glove
(Fig. 4.21B).

2. Place the thumb of the ungloved hand
between the wrist and cuff on the gloved hand and
carefully pull off the glove (Fig. 4.21C). Finally, dispose of the gloves in the appropriate container.

5

Office surgery using the 'non-touch' technique

Although it is not the intention of this book to explain operative techniques in any detail nevertheless two procedures are explained here because both are common to almost all podiatrists, podiatric students and assistants. These are the avulsion of toe nails and the treatment of warts (verrucae).

Because these two procedures are commonly performed in an office environment/surgery, as opposed to that of the operating room, they have been included to show the role of both the assistant and podiatrist using a technique often referred to as the 'non-touch technique'. In this technique, although the basic rules of the sterile surgical field are maintained, the 'full' operating room procedures for draping and gowning are not used. For instance, patients remain in their outer clothes, and the surgeon and assistant wear either scrub suits or white office coats over their normal clothing.

TOTAL NAIL AVULSION: THE PHENOL–ALCOHOL TECHNIQUE

Whilst the podiatrist is carrying out the preoperative assessment, the patient having signed the consent form, you as the assistant can prepare the instrument trolley.

The following items are required for all nail procedures (i.e. part or total avulsion) (see Fig. 5.1):

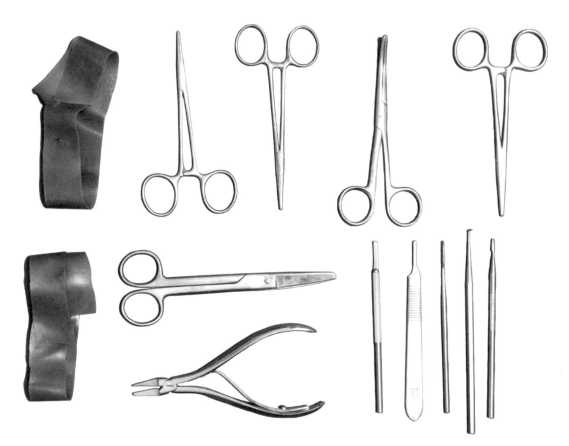

Figure 5.1 Nail avulsion basic pack. (Reproduced with permission from the Department of Medical Illustration, Ipswich Hospital NHS Trust, Ipswich, UK.)

- no. 3 scalpel handle (1)
- no. 15 scalpel blade (1)
- haemostat, straight (2)
- toothed dissecting forceps (1)
- nail elevator (1)
- nail splitter (or a Beaver handle with a 62 blade) (1)
- Blacks file (1)
- mosquito haemostat (1)
- Thwaites nail nippers (1)
- dressing scissors (1)
- phenol applicator/orange sticks (wooden) (3)
- Penrose tourniquet (1)
- non-stick dressings (1 per toe)
- outer dressings (as required)
- Tubinette® size 12 (as required)
- local anaesthetic (as required)
- aspirating syringe (1)

- syringe needle 27 g (1)
- liquefied phenol 80–88%
- foot preparation disinfectant (e.g. Betadine®)
- sterile swabs (as required)
- outer dressing adhesive plasters (as required)
- isopropyl alcohol 70% (flush)
- sterile foot drape (1 per foot)
- alcohol foot wash (e.g. Hibitane® in 70% IMS)

Setting out the trolley

Having cleaned the trolley top with an alcohol wipe, you should now lay a waterproof paper towel over the trolley. These towels normally come in sterile packs. You must therefore hold only the edges of the towel, taking care not to touch its inner surface or centre.

> **NOTE:** This towel once placed on the trolley should no longer be considered sterile.

Next drop a folded sterile green drape on to the centre of the waterproof cover, with the folds of the drape *uppermost*. Again, touch only the outer corners of the green drape, and take care not to touch the inner surface. Allow the drape to unfold and fall around the edges of the trolley. You may then 'drop' non-delicate instruments and dressings on to the draped trolley.

Alternatively, and by far the better method, wait until the podiatrist is wearing sterile gloves and then present the instruments and dressings (as explained on p. 31 and in Fig. 2.10).

It is of course not unusual for podiatrists working in their office to use hospital prepacked nail avulsion instrument packs, in which case the instrument pack will be opened by the podiatrist wearing sterile surgical gloves (as explained on p. 45 and in Fig. 3.7). You will have first opened the outer cover.

Administration of the local anaesthetic

> **CAUTION:** Do not use an anaesthetic that has a vasoconstrictor agent, such as epinephrine (adrenaline). This could in some instances lead to necrosis of the digit.

Having assessed the patient and cleaned the intended injection site with an appropriate alcohol wipe (e.g. Hibitane® in 70% IMS) the podiatrist (wearing non-sterile gloves) will then administer the local anaesthetic. If prilocaine 4% (plain) is used, normally only one 2.2 ml cartridge will be required.

> **TIP:** Don't forget to take the patient's blood pressure before administering the anaesthetic.

Although an adequate field block can normally be achieved by injecting only the medial and lateral aspects of the toe, sometimes the distal end of the toe is found to be still sensitive to touch some time after the administration of the anaesthetic. In these instances the medial and lateral plantar nerves may have been missed. The problem can be avoided if you apply the injection to each aspect of the toe (total block) (Fig. 5.2).

> **TIP:** When injecting the anaesthetic ensure that the needle point does not penetrate the matrix area, or the nail sulci, as it is possible for the phenol to filter into the needle tracts and cause a chemical burn at the injection site (postphenol epidermoid cyst).

Preoperative foot wash

> **TIP:** Whether the whole foot or only the toe needs to be washed by you will depend on the protocol of the department that you are working in.

The podiatrist will now have gloved with sterile surgical gloves, using the open-glove method (as shown on p. 42 and in Fig. 3.5). You are now free to hand the podiatrist the required instruments and the foot drape. This foot drape is generally made of cloth and covers the foot to above

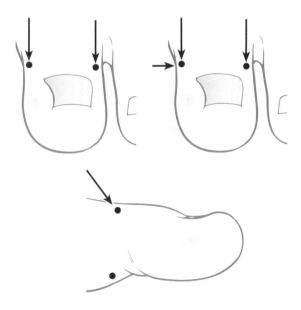

Figure 5.2 Injection sites for TNA.

the ankle. There is normally a manufactured aperture for the toe. A sterile paper or cloth towel may also be used as a foot drape to wrap around the foot and ankle, leaving the toe free.

The podiatrist places the drape over the foot, taking care not to allow the gloved hands to touch the patient (including the toe). With the patient's toe now protruding through the aperture, either you or the podiatrist can then paint the toe with an antiseptic preoperative paint (such as Betadine®).

The podiatrist now applies the Penrose tourniquet. This tourniquet can come in various forms, from a simple rubber tube to a commercially manufactured one. Often, in practice, a thin rubber strip approximately 20 cm (8″) long by 1.5 cm ($\frac{3}{4}$″) wide is used. This is applied to the tip of the toe and then wound back to the base so as to exsanguinate the toe, where it is held in place by a haemostat.

TIP: The Penrose tourniquet must be tagged or a haemostat used so that there can be no possibility of the patient accidentally leaving the procedure room with the tourniquet still in place, with obvious disastrous results.

Do not use the rim on the cuff of a surgical glove as a tourniquet! These have been known to have been accidentally left in place.

Total nail avulsion (TNA)

The podiatrist will first confirm that the toe is adequately anaesthetized. If there is profuse granulation tissue present (Fig. 5.3A) then a scalpel handle with a no. 15 blade attached will be taken. Using sharp dissection the podiatrist will then remove the granulation tissue in total (Fig. 5.3B). In a badly swollen toe this procedure looks (to students) excessively severe. However, the sharply cut edges normally heal very quickly, whereas leaving the granulation tissue in place can in some instances prolong the postoperative healing time.

TIP: Silver nitrate is occasionally used to reduce small areas of granulation tissue when the partial nail avulsion technique is used. In this case care

---

must be taken to avoid the silver nitrate touching the nail, as it may cause erosions on the edge of the nail leading to possible postoperative complications.

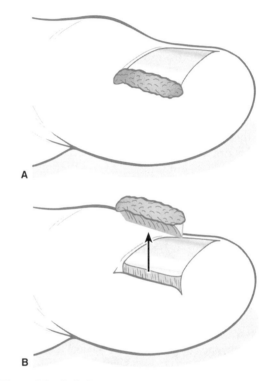

Figure 5.3   A, B: Excision of granulation tissue.

Removing the nail plate

Although various methods are employed for this, the procedure explained here is one I have used with excellent results on many hundreds of nails.

First a nail elevator (Fig. 5.4) is used. The podiatrist slips the edge of the elevator under the eponychium (unguinal fold) on either the medial or lateral side of the nail plate (depending on whether the surgeon is right or left handed, also which foot is being operated on). Right-handed surgeons tend to start on the lateral aspect on the left foot and the medial aspect on the right foot.

The elevator is inserted only sufficiently to allow the tip of the instrument to rupture the tissue and is then moved from side to side.

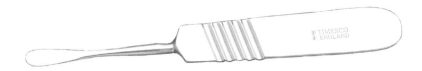

Figure 5.4 Nail elevator. (Reproduced with permission from Timesco Surgical & Medical, London, UK.)

Secondly on the (right foot, with a right-handed surgeon) the elevator is inserted under the nail plate on the medial side of the nail (Fig. 5.5). While pressing with the thumb on the lateral side of the toe the podiatrist now brings the blade of the elevator towards the thumb in a single peeling motion. This should separate the nail plate from the bed. The loosened nail is then held by a haemostat and extracted with a slight twist. Any nail and loose tissue debris on the nail bed should then be removed using the Blacks file, before applying the phenol.

> **TIP:** Inspect the proximal edge of the nail plate to see if it is smooth; if it is not there is the possibility that a fragment of the nail has been left in place. This must be removed.

A white crescent-shaped area is found at the base of the nail (the lunula). Occasionally this may be loose at its distal edge. If loose the podiatrist may consider it preferable to remove this, in which case the tissue can be held by toothed dissecting forceps. (If it is not loose it is left in place.)

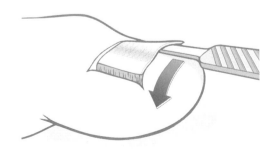

Figure 5.5 Nail avulsion.

> **TIP:** A haemostat may be used in this instance as the tissue is going to be removed, but remember a haemostat must not be used on tissue that is to be preserved.

The podiatrist now holds the dissecting forceps in a pincer grip, raises the distal edge of the lunula (Fig. 5.6) and, using the 15 blade, carefully excises the complete wedge of tissue.

> **TIP:** After the excision of the lunula, when the tourniquet is removed there is often considerably more bleeding than would be expected from a normal nail avulsion. Therefore a pressure bandage should be applied for at least 5 minutes, preferably with the foot elevated.

Application of the phenol

> **CAUTION:** When applying the phenol it is advisable that both the assistant and podiatrist wear gloves and some form of eye protection.

The method for applying the phenol differs from school to school and from clinic to clinic. One accepted method is to use wooden applicators, known as orange sticks. Some have cotton-wool tips; I prefer to use an orange stick without the cotton wool, in which case three sticks are used. Each applicator is dipped into *fresh* phenol.

> **TIP:** Try not to get too much phenol on the applicator tip, and do not flick excess phenol off the applicator.

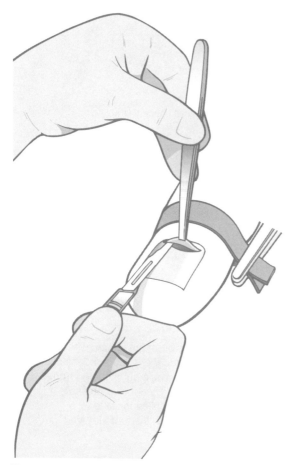

Figure 5.6 Removing the lunula.

The phenol is applied by the podiatrist to the nail groove and matrix area. This is done for 1 minute then, with a new applicator, the procedure is repeated for a minute, and again with the third applicator the procedure is repeated for a further minute.

> **TIP:** Do not reuse the applicator if a 'frequent-use bottle' is used to store the phenol. A fresh applicator must be used each time.

When the podiatrist has finished applying the phenol, you can now copiously flush the surgical site with isopropyl alcohol.

The tourniquet is now released and the dressings applied. On average the total tourniquet time for this procedure is 5 minutes. *In any event do not leave the tourniquet on for more than 20 minutes.*

When the podiatrist is satisfied that there is no noticeable postoperative bleeding the inner dressings are applied. You can now hand the podiatrist the outer dressing.

> **TIP:** If this is a size 12 Tubinette®, for a bulky dressing the length required is approximately from your finger tips to your elbow. To cover a smaller dressing the length required is approximately three times the length of the toe.

> **TIP:** Phenol may be supplied in 8 ml 'frequent-use bottles'. For satisfactory results the phenol must be fresh. Fresh phenol is clear or has a light pink colour. If it is dark or brown it should not be used. The date that the bottle was opened should be entered on the label. If the bottle has been opened and there is no date shown DO NOT USE IT. If a 'frequent-use bottle' is used this should be replaced after 1 month.
> Fresh phenol will also immediately blanch the skin.

There are a number of other nail avulsion techniques used, although most appear to have now fallen out of favour. The student podiatrist may nevertheless like to read the appropriate literature and compare the more common alternative procedures, which are: the DuVries, Winograd, Frost, Zadik, and Kaplan techniques.

Partial nail avulsion (PNA)

The preparation of the toe is almost the same as that for the TNA. However, in this instance only the edge of the nail plate and matrix are removed.

Using a Thwaites nail cutter (Fig. 5.7) the podiatrist positions the tip of the cutter approximately 0.3 cm ($\frac{1}{8}''$) from the medial or lateral edge, depending on which edge is ingrowing. Taking care not to prise the nail plate from the nail beds the anvil blade of the cutter is gently

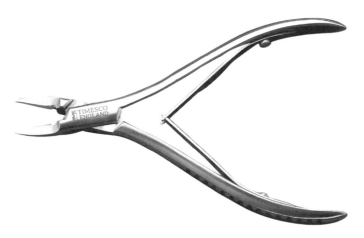

Figure 5.7   Thwaites nail cutter. (Reproduced with permission from Timesco Surgical & Medical, London, UK.)

forced under the nail. When in position the cutting edge is lowered to split the nail.

Having split the distal portion of the nail the podiatrist inserts a nail splitter (Fig. 5.8) or a no. 62 Beaver blade. With this the split distal to proximal beneath the eponychium can be lengthened (this can be felt as a slight 'give' as the nail splitter goes through the matrix). The offending nail spicule is now excised by clamping it with a mosquito haemostat and gently removing it in a twisting motion. The twist is towards the remaining nail plate.

> **TIP:** When using the nail splitter, try to split the nail by following the linear nail lines.

Postoperative advice

As well as the standard postoperative advice given for any surgical case it may be prudent to advise the patient that there may be a slight discharge from the wound, and that this may continue for up to 6 weeks.

There is also a possibility that at approximately 8 to 12 days after surgery there may be a noticeable discharge. Advise patients that this is not an infection but the result of the phenol application, but if they are in any way concerned about it that they should return to have the wound examined.

> **TIP:** Patients should also be made aware, preferably in writing, that there is the possibility of the nail regrowing, irrespective of what method was used.

Antibiotics are rarely required after nail surgery, with the possible exception of patients who have surgical prosthesis (hip, knee, etc.) or a history of rheumatic fever.

> **CAUTION:** Phenol is a corrosive acid. If phenol is accidentally spilt over the skin, the area must be washed with copious amounts of water or olive oil. A small spill on the toe should be wiped off with glycerin. If phenol enters the eye, this

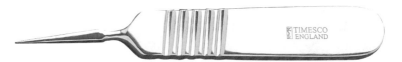

Figure 5.8   Nail splitter. (Reproduced with permission from Timesco Surgical & Medical, London, UK.)

must be flushed with water and the casualty transported to the hospital emergency department at once. If possible, continue to flush the eye whilst the casualty is being taken to the emergency room. Remove contaminated clothing instantly.

TREATMENT FOR A WART (VERRUCA)

There are almost as many ways of treating a verruca as there are podiatrists treating them, and most podiatrists have their favourite depending on their success rate. These treatments are for the most part chemical. The more common ones are as follows:

- *chemical* treatments including:
  —5% formaldehyde
  —monochloracetic acid
  —nitric acid
  —pyrogallic acid
  —salicylic acid
  —silver nitrate

  —trichloracetic acid
- *cryosurgery* (the use of extreme cold to freeze and destroy tissue):
  —carbon dioxide gas
  —liquid nitrogen
- *surgery*:
  —curettage
  —surgical excision
- *electrosurgery*:
  —fulguration
  —electrodesiccation
  —biactive coagulation.

We are going to look in detail at a procedure known as fulguration, although this may also sometimes be known as hyfrecation as the machine used may be a Conmed Hyfrecator® (Fig. 5.9).

NOTE: Basically fulguration means the destruction of tissue by means of high-frequency electric sparks. It should not be confused with electrosection where the current used is designed for cutting.

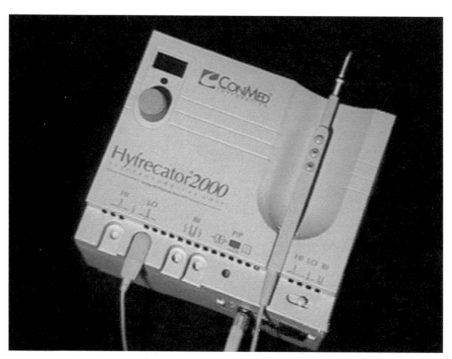

Figure 5.9   Conmed Hyfrecator Model 2000®. (Photograph courtesy of Schuco International London Ltd.)

> **CAUTION:** In view of the electric charge employed in fulguration it may be considered advisable not to use this form of treatment on the following patients: patients with heart pacemakers, with a metal prosthesis, who suffer from epilepsy or who are very nervous.

Equipment required includes the following:

- Conmed Hyfrecator® (or similar equipment)
- no. 3 scalpel handle (1)
- no. 11 scalpel blade (1)
- local anaesthetic (as required)
- aspirating syringe (1)
- 27 g syringe needle (1)
- toothed dissecting forceps (1)
- dressings (as required).

After you have confirmed that the patient is a suitable candidate for this form of treatment, the patient should sign a consent form. You should also check the patient's blood pressure at this point.

> **TIP:** Advise the patient of the possibility of scar formation. On rare occasions the formation of a scar can cause more problems in the long term than the original verruca.

> **CAUTION:** If the foot or the site is to be washed do not use alcohol or other flammable cleansing agents. This is because of the risk of fire when the Hyfrecator® is discharged.

Although some people can tolerate fulguration without anaesthesia it is probably prudent, unless the verruca is exceedingly small, to use a local anaesthetic. Use only a small amount; 0.5 ml of prilocaine 4% under the verruca is usually sufficient. If the verruca is *not* on a toe then a vasoconstrictor can be added to the anaesthetic (1:100 000 epinephrine).

Procedure

The trolley is prepared as for a nail avulsion. The podiatrist ensures that the verruca is suitably anaesthetized, and then places the electrode slightly above and close to the verruca. The current is then applied.

> **TIP:** Make sure that you, the podiatrist and the patient are not touching any metal object. If you find that you are touching a metal object whilst using the equipment you should not let go and retouch the object again whilst the equipment is discharging, or you may get a shock. This also applies if you are touching the patient's foot with your hand.

It is important that the point of the needle (the electrode) is positioned close to the verruca, so that the spark from the needle may be applied over the surface of the verruca until it is blanched. Some podiatrists may alternatively penetrate the verruca with the needle tip, then give two or three short applications. The amount and depth of tissue that can be destroyed by each application is generally dependent on the following:

- current setting
- length of time of the application (current flowing)
- density of the tissue and its moisture content
- distance between the electrode and the tissue
- type of electrode used.

> **TIP:** If the electrode is too far from the verruca the electrical arc that is formed may be diverted to adjacent tissue. This also occurs if the skin is wet.

Tissue destruction is characterized by the formation of an eschar. A no. 11 scalpel blade is now taken to excise the burnt tissue. If care is used the verruca can be removed completely with no haemorrhaging. Some podiatrists prefer to remove the verruca with a curette (Fig. 5.10) after fulguration.

If the verruca is left in place after fulguration a liquefaction necrosis usually occurs 8 to 10 days later. The verruca can be evacuated at this time. Also, if the verruca is on the dorsal surface of a

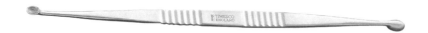

Figure 5.10 Volkmann oval double-ended curette. (Reproduced with permission from Timesco Surgical & Medical, London, UK.)

toe there is often no need to remove it after fulguration as the scab drops off after about 6 days, leaving healthy skin.

Postoperative considerations

After fulguration the healing time for small lesions is approximately 3 weeks, with healing by second intention (i.e. granulation from the base). On rare occasions the granulation forms at the top of the wound instead of the base. There may then be severe pain if the lesion is on a weight-bearing area. If so, it will have to be opened for drainage.

If the area is large (which is to be avoided if possible) the wound will heal by third intention. This generally results in the formation of a scar.

A small lesion on a non-weight-bearing surface may only require a Band-Aid® or similar dressing. However, a lesion on a weight-bearing area may require the use of a 5 mm felt cavity pad. As in any surgical procedure you should take care to prevent secondary infection. The patient should be given postoperative care instructions.

6

After surgery

POSTOPERATIVE PATIENT CARE

After the procedure the patient may be transferred to the postoperative recovery room, staying there for a period of at least half an hour before being discharged home in the company of a responsible adult.

During the transfer from the operating room the sides of the patient's trolley must be in the 'up' position, and the patient may be given a blanket if required, although the foot that was operated on should not be covered.

The nurse or assistant receiving the patient must check that the correct documentation has travelled with the patient, with particular attention to any postoperative instructions that the podiatrist has given.

If the patient is to remain on the trolley the foot-end of the trolley should be elevated at least 15 cm, to assist in postoperative haemorrhage control. Then, depending on local protocol, the patient's vital signs may be recorded in the patient's notes.

> **TIP:** The patient should be left unattended only if there is access to a nurse call system.

The patient may also be given some form of pain-killing medication (before the local anaesthetic has worn off), with a further supply to take home.

TIP: Before giving the patient any medication in tablet form, check whether the patient can swallow tablets whole, or if tablets in a dissolvable form are needed.

The dressing must be inspected within the first 10 minutes to check whether any noticeable postoperative haemorrhaging has occurred. If there is and the bloodstain is wider than 2 cm it may be advisable to continue to monitor the dressing for a further 5 minutes. If the stain is no wider after that time then the outer dressing can be changed, but the inner dressing should be left undisturbed. If there has been significant bleeding—for example, a stain of over 5 cm in diameter developing within 10 minutes—the podiatrist must be informed, and the wound inspected.

POSTOPERATIVE X-RAY

TIP: If fixation screws or K wires have been employed it is advisable to have the foot X-rayed before the patient leaves the department. The rationale for this is that if at a later date the patient has an accident that results in the pin being dislodged then you will be able to demonstrate that the pin and toe were in correct alignment when the patient was discharged.

ADVICE TO THE PATIENT ON NORMAL POSTOPERATIVE OBSERVATIONS

Before discharging patients they should be reminded of the normal postoperative observations such as the following.

- They may notice a certain degree of swelling in or around the surgical site, and this may take a number of weeks to subside totally.
- They may experience a sudden sharp stabbing pain that lasts for about a second every now and again, and that this may continue for a number of weeks after surgery.
- After the sutures have been removed and baths are allowed they may notice that the surgical site will become red or purple. This can continue for some weeks after surgery.
- After bunion surgery they may find that for a number of weeks they are walking on the outer border of their foot.

The patient should also be advised to contact the department or return if any of the following occur:

- there is any marked increase in pain
- if a bloodstain of over 2 cm in diameter appears on the dressing
- if the dressing appears to be excessively tight
- if pain is experienced in the thigh, back of the lower leg or chest
- if the dressing accidentally gets wet or excessively dirty
- if there is loss of sensation in the foot or toe, or the foot feels cold or very hot
- if in any doubt about anything.

TIP: Always give the patient a contact telephone number.

Resting after surgery

Because severe pain is uncommon after forefoot podiatric surgery the patient may underestimate the need to rest. Patients should therefore be firmly advised that failure to rest can result in a very painful and swollen toe.

POSTOPERATIVE FOOTWEAR

In outpatient podiatric forefoot surgery patients usually have the foot bandaged, and the patient wears a postoperative surgical shoe (Fig. 6.1) as opposed to a plaster cast. If a fixation pin has been

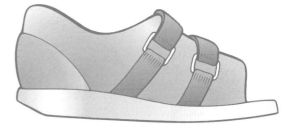

Figure 6.1 Postoperative surgical shoe.

used the patient should therefore be advised that the surgical shoe needs to be worn for at least 6 weeks postoperatively and also that it must be worn every time that the foot is put to the floor.

WALKING STICKS

Because the majority of forefoot surgical procedures allow the patient to bear weight after surgery, walking sticks are often employed. The stick must be of the correct length, and to find this length two common methods are used. The first, and probably the commoner, is to measure the distance from the crease on the wrist, with the patient standing in shoes and the elbow flexed about 10–15° to the ground. The second method is to measure the distance from the greater trochanter to the ground.

TIP: The walking stick should be held on the opposite side to the affected foot.

Advise the patient that the gait sequence is to advance the stick on the unaffected side and the affected foot simultaneously, and then advance the unaffected foot in front of the affected foot.

IMPORTANT TIP: Telephone the patient the next day, or at least within the first 24 hours after surgery, to ask how the patient is or if there are any queries. Postoperative attentiveness is very important for avoiding misunderstandings and possible litigation.

7

Suturing

As a podiatric surgical assistant, unless you are a surgical pupil, you will not normally be expected to carry out any suturing unless you have had extensive advanced training and local protocol allows it. Nevertheless it is essential that you are aware of the different types of suture material and suturing techniques that are used.

> **TIP:** If you are a surgical pupil then in your early days it is essential that you practise your suturing on a daily basis, and then practise some more. A pig's trotter is an ideal object for practising incisions and suturing techniques.

Something that tends to be forgotten is that the postoperative scar can be seen as the 'surgeon's signature' and if you work regularly with a group of surgeons you will soon find that you can tell who has performed the operation, or at least applied the sutures, solely by the appearance of the scar. The scar is also what the patient sees and shows to others.

> **TIP:** With a few exceptions, keloid scarring for example, the appearance of the scar is largely dependent on the neatness of the suturing. So if when you are suturing you do not like the positioning of your suture, remove it and do it again.

SUTURES AND LIGATURES

The difference between a suture and a ligature is as follows.

Sutures. A suture is a stitch used to approximate the tissue or structures until the healing process is complete.

Ligatures. A ligature is a suture that is used to encircle a blood vessel to arrest bleeding.

SUTURE AND LIGATURE SIZES COMMONLY USED IN PODIATRIC SURGERY

Suture and ligature material come in various sizes. The method of expressing the size is the same for all sutures and ligatures. For example, a suture package may be marked as [2 (3/0)]; the first number, 2, refers to the metric gauge; the number in parentheses, 3/0, refers to the old equivalent thread size denoted by the USP (United States Pharmacopeia) or BPC (British Pharmacopoeia) standard ranges. This is the system most commonly used in practice and will be used in this text. The range of sizes available is shown in Table 7.1.

> **TIP:** The lower the number the deeper the suture is placed in the wound. For instance, normally a 2/0 would be placed deeper than a 3/0.

CATEGORIES OF SUTURE AND LIGATURE MATERIALS

Both ligatures and sutures are divided into two principal groups: absorbable and non-absorbable.

Absorbable sutures are, as the name implies, absorbed or dissolved into the tissues by hydrolysis during the healing process. In some cases they take up to 2 months to dissolve.

Non-absorbable sutures will, on the other hand, remain permanently within the tissue after the healing process is completed. In podiatric surgery this type would normally be a metallic wire. The other common non-absorbable sutures that are used for skin closure may be made of some form of nylon or polyester.

Both absorbable and non-absorbable sutures may be made of either natural or synthetic material:

Table 7.1 Suture sizes

USP/BPC	Metric
11/0	0.1
10/0	0.2
9/0	0.3
8/0	0.4
7/0	0.5
6/0*	**0.75***
5/0*	**1.0***
4/0*	**1.5***
3/0*	**2.0***
2/0*	**2.5***
0*	**3.0***
1	4.0
2	5.0
3	6.0

* Thread sizes regularly used in podiatric surgery ranging from thinnest to thickest: 0.75 (6/0) : 1 (5/0) : 1.5 (4/0) : 2 (3/0) : 2.5 (2/0) : 3 (0).

- *absorbable*:
  - —natural: catgut, collagen
  - —synthetic: polyglycolic acid
- *non-absorbable*:
  - —natural: silk, linen, cotton
  - —synthetic: polyesters, polyamides, polyoletins, metallic wire, metal suture clips.

SUTURES

Absorbable sutures

One of the commonest absorbable sutures used in podiatric surgery is Dexon®, a synthetic polymer of glycolic acid, which is absorbed in the tissues by hydrolysis. The sizes normally used in podiatric surgery are: 2/0 for closing joint capsules, 3/0 for approximating the individual skin layers and 4/0 for subcuticular skin closure. Sizes 4/0 and 3/0 are also commonly used for ligatures. The time of minimal absorption in the tissues is approximately 15 days, that of maximum absorption is approximately 30 days and complete absorption occurs between 60 and 80 days after insertion.

> **TIP:** Individual surgeons may have different preferred suture sizes for the same tissue.

Another common synthetic absorbable suture used in podiatric surgery is Vicryl®. It is generally used in sizes of 0, 2/0, and 3/0 for capsule and deep tissue repairs. These are also polyglycolic acid sutures. They are extremely inert and cause minimal tissue reaction. Because they are fray resistant they do not become slippery when used.

Non-absorbable sutures

The Ethilon® range of non-absorbable sutures is probably the most commonly used in podiatric surgery for wound closure. Sizes range from 3/0 to 6/0. They are made of monofilament polyamide, and are generally blue in colour. The 3/0 size in conjunction with a reverse cutting curved 19 mm needle is used for external skin closure; the material length in this combination is approximately 45 cm.

> **TIP:** Any non-absorbable sutures that are braided should generally not be used in an infected wound as it is possible that this may lead to a sinus formation. In the presence of a known infection a single-strand nylon suture, which is relatively inert, may be used instead with relative safety.

Polypropylene

Monofilament polypropylene sutures, often the 2/0 size (which is deep blue in colour), are also popular in podiatric surgery. They are used for capsule closures and tendon repair, being both extremely inert and stronger than monofilament nylon.

Metallic wire

Metallic surgical wire is occasionally used in some bunion procedures. Wires are generally made of stainless steel, tantalum or silver, and can come as a single-strand wire or as a multifilament wire. The latter is the more flexible, although care needs to be taken to avoid kinking the wire.

Sizes are normally graded as SWG (standard wire gauge) and range from (fine) 40 SWG up to (stout) 18 SWG . Wire of sizes 29 to 18 SWG may be used for wiring bone.

> **TIP:** A very important consideration when using metallic sutures or wires is to ensure that wires of different metals do not come into contact with each other in the tissues, otherwise corrosion is likely to occur.

Metal sutures (staples)

These are only occasionally used in podiatric surgery. They have two sharp points, which, when the clip is closed, grip the edges of the skin incision together (Fig. 7.1). They are not suitable for closure of deep wounds. The sutures are fastened with a staple gun, and are removed at the same time as normal external sutures. (The average is 14 days for the foot.)

ADHESIVE SKIN CLOSURES

Adhesive skin closures such as Steristrips® are widely used, often in conjunction with a subcuticular skin closure, to give added support to the suture. Adhesion to the skin may be increased by applying a thin coating of 'plastic skin'—Opsite® (see Fig. 4.19A, p. 63) or Tincture Benz®—to each side of the wound. These come as sprays, but the substance should not be sprayed directly on the wound, as this can delay epithelialization. Instead spray the coating

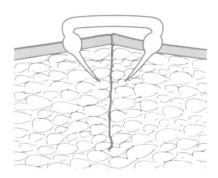

Figure 7.1 Staple in position.

on to a swab and than dab this around the wound. After this, apply one end of the Steristrip® and gently bring the edges together before positioning the other end (see Fig. 4.19B, p. 63).

Superglue (Histoacryl®)

The use of a 'superglue' is uncommon in podiatry, with the possible exception of closing heel fissures. In use the key point is that the *glue is not placed in the wound*, but rather should be used to bond the edges of the wound together. The skin edges are opposed and the glue is put on to the surface of the wound edges in a line of 'spot welds'. The edges should then be held together for 30 seconds after the application to allow the glue to set.

> **TIP:** You must not use a non-medically approved commercial superglue.

LIGATURES

You will on occasion be asked to assist in the fastening of a ligature, often around the end of a blood vessel to close the lumen. Normally an absorbable suture, often size 3/0 or 4/0 Dexon®, will be used. The podiatrist will clamp the end of the vessel with artery forceps. At this stage you may be asked to take the handle of the forceps, as the podiatrist passes one end of the ligature from one hand to the other so that the thread is held behind the forceps, then allows the thread to drop around the blood vessel. At this point you may be asked to depress the forceps blade to lift the blood vessel as the knot is made, with the podiatrist taking care to avoid tying in the tip of the artery forceps (see Fig. 4.12, p. 58). If the forceps are trapped by the ligature, the latter will be pulled off the blood vessel as the forceps are removed. As the podiatrist tightens the knot you will be asked to slightly relax the grip of the forceps tip, but *you must not remove the forceps completely* until the ligature is secure.

> **TIP:** Take care that you do not cut the thread too near the knot.

LOADING NEEDLES

In your role as scrub assistant you will be expected to load needles on to the needle holder. Experience will tell you which needle size and suture material will be required for a specific task. In all cases you should avoid handling the needle more than is necessary. As detailed in Chapter 4, remember to keep the needle holder at right angles to the curve of the needle, and just to one side of the half-way point of the curve towards the thread end (Fig. 7.2A). This will allow the podiatrist to manoeuvre the curve of the needle through the tissues. If the needle holder is too near the point the podiatrist will find it impossible to pass the needle through the tissue; if too near the thread end, as well as being unstable it may well break or the thread come off (Fig. 7.2B).

> **TIP:** Don't forget, when loading needle holders for left-handed surgeons the point of the needle as mounted on the needle holder will be in the opposite direction to that for right-handed surgeons.

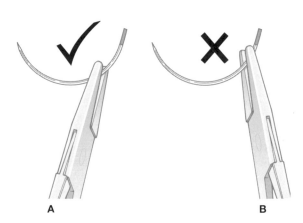

A　　　　　　　　　　　　　　　**B**

Figure 7.2 A: Correct and B: incorrect position for the needle holder.

SUTURING METHODS EMPLOYED IN PODIATRIC SURGERY

Tying the knot

Practice in knot tying is essential in your early days. There are three basic knots employed in surgery: the square knot often referred to as a reef knot (Fig. 7.3A), the surgeon's knot (Fig. 7.3B) and the nylon knot (Fig. 7.3C). A further knot that is often the result of an incorrectly attempted square knot is the granny knot (Fig. 7.3D); in this knot the ends of the threads are not parallel but instead alternate, one being first over and then under the other (see diagram). The result of this is that the knot will probably slip under tension.

The hand tie

By far the most useful hand-tied knot in podiatric surgery is the square knot. As this knot holds well it is suitable for deep wounds that are difficult to close with an instrument tie.

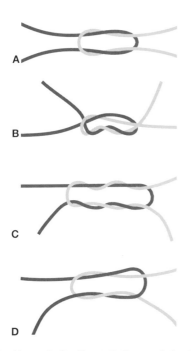

Figure 7.3   Knots. A: Reef knot. B: Surgeon's knot. C: Nylon knot. D: Granny knot.

Method. Take one end of the thread in each hand then pass the *right* end over the left end. Tighten this to make a simple knot. Next pass the *left* end over the right, then tighten to complete the knot.

Some general considerations when knot tying include the following.

- The knot should be as small as possible. If the knot is tied correctly then placing extra throws will not add strength to the knot but only increase its bulk.
- When hand tying, during positioning of the suture try to avoid a sawing motion as this could cause friction between the strands as you form the knot.
- Avoid excessive tension, as this may result in the suture snapping or in tearing of the tissue.
- When suturing for approximation the suture should not be tied too tightly, as this may contribute to tissue strangulation.
- After the first throw it is necessary to maintain a slight pull on one end of the thread as you form the second throw. This is especially important if the knot is going to be under any tension from the tissues, as failure to maintain tension with the first throw will result in a loose knot.
- To form a good flat knot the final tension on the final throw should be as nearly horizontal as possible.

If you are not happy with the suture then remove it and try again.

The instrument tie

By far the commonest way to tie knots is the instrument tie. This is performed as follows.

Method. Having pulled the thread through the tissues (from right to left if a right-handed person) leave a short 'tail'. Then take the long end of the thread with the needle attached in your left hand, with the needle holder still in your right hand (Fig. 7.4).

> **TIP:** Beginners may find it easier when using a needle holder to grasp the short tail of the suture with forceps. This avoids accidentally pulling the suture through completely with the left hand.

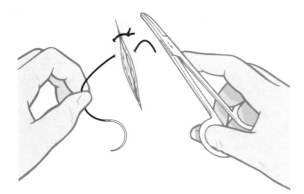

Figure 7.4 Leaving a short tail.

Then, holding your left hand in the same position, press the needle holder against the thread (Fig. 7.5). Take care not to allow the short end to slip through the wound.

> **TIP:** Some surgeons may rotate the shaft of the needle holder around the thread, as opposed to wrapping the thread around the needle holder. It is suggested that you adopt the method that you find the easiest.

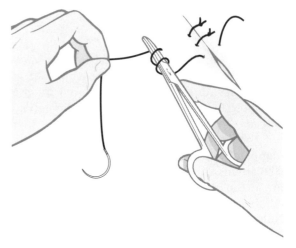

Figure 7.6 Wrapping the thread twice around the needle holder.

Still pressing the needle holder against the thread, with the left hand wrap the thread *twice* around the needle holder (Fig. 7.6).

Then take hold of the short end with tips of the needle holder and pull the throws down to the short end (Fig. 7.7).

At this stage the left hand goes to the right, and the right hand goes to the left (crossing hands) (Fig. 7.8). This will make the knot 'lie flat' and the short end (held in the needle holder) will now be to the left of the incision. When in place, release the short end of the thread.

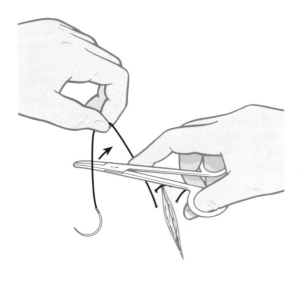

Figure 7.5 Pressing the needle holder against the thread.

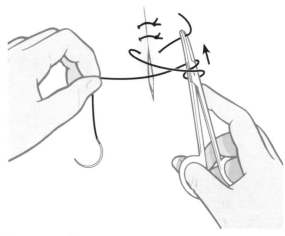

Figure 7.7 Sliding the thread down to the short tail.

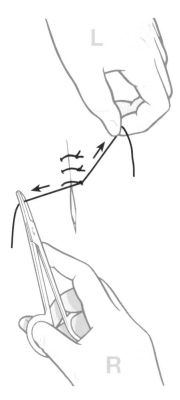

Figure 7.8 Crossing hands.

Keeping the needle holder in the same position (i.e. hands still crossed), bring the left hand (which is still holding the needle end of the thread) across to the left. This will bring the thread against the needle holder. Now make *one* wrap around the needle holder in the opposite direction to the first. Pull this wrap down to the first knot. Pull the left hand to the left, and the right to the right; this will cause the knot to lie squarely. You should then put at least one further throw on the knot. The thread should be cut approximately 0.5 cm from the knot, although with a nylon thread, which may slip, it may be advisable to leave the end slightly longer.

TIP: Sutures should be cut so that ends are shorter than the distance between adjacent sutures, to avoid entanglement.

Interrupted (simple) sutures

Often known as 'simples', as the name suggests, in this type each stitch is tied separately (Fig. 7.9A). This allows the removal of one or more of the sutures without disturbing the whole wound. (Occasionally removal is required if the wound becomes infected, or if a suture was incorrectly placed.)

Method. To do a simple suture the podiatrist will position the needle so that equal 'bites' of tissue can be taken from each side (Fig. 7.9B). Although the actual distance between the needle insertion and the wound edge, and also the distance between the individual stitches, is to some extent dependent on the skin thickness as well as the area being sutured, generally the distance between individual sutures along the length of the wound is about 4 to 5 mm.

The distance between the needle entry point and the edge of the wound must be the same as the distance between the needle exit point and wound edge (Fig. 7.9C). Therefore, the deeper the wound the greater should be the distance from the wound edge to the needle entry point, equally the depth of the needle bite will be deeper (Fig. 7.9D).

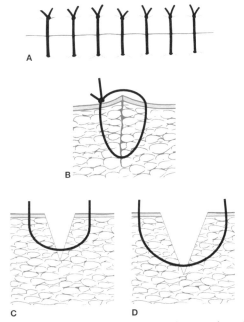

Figure 7.9 A, B: Simple sutures. C, D: Distance from the edge is dependent on depth.

Care should be taken to ensure that the wound edges approximate without inversion or overlap and, importantly, without excessive tension.

> **TIP:** A tight knot on a loose suture is basically the idea, as the suture will tighten with the postoperative swelling.

Too tight a suture could well result in necrosis of the wound edges or tearing of the skin. Toothed dissecting forceps are held on one side of the wound to evert and stabilize the edge of the wound as the needle is positioned, although occasionally both sides of the wound may be held together. In either case the needle enters the skin on the first side at an angle of 90° to the skin surface (Fig. 7.10).

Equal amounts of tissue are included on both sides of the wound edges so that the angle of exit of the needle on the opposite incision edge will be the same as that of the entrance.

> **TIP:** In areas of delicate skin, skin (Gillies) hooks (Fig. 7.11) may be used to evert the skin. Alternatively, fine toothed dissecting forceps (Adson's) (Fig. 7.12) may be applied to the inner layer of dermis.

In some instances it may be advisable to pass through the edges of the wound one at a time. In this case the needle is passed through the first side of the wound, and taken out of the wound, then is re-entered into the wound and passed through the second side (Fig. 7.13). It is tied in the normal manner.

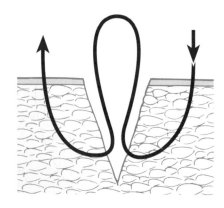

Figure 7.13   In-and-out method for deep simple sutures.

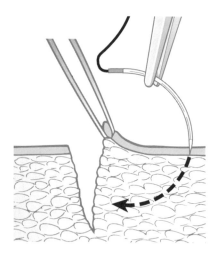

Figure 7.10   Entry at 90° to the skin.

Figure 7.11   Gillies skin hook. (Reproduced with permission from Timesco Surgical & Medical, London, UK.)

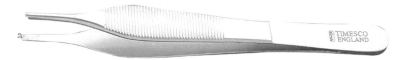

Figure 7.12   Adson's forceps. (Reproduced with permission from Timesco Surgical & Medical, London, UK.

Mattress sutures

Horizontal mattress sutures

These are often used in place of simple sutures and are basically two simple sutures in one. They give good skin apposition with cosmetic scar line comparable to that of simple sutures (Fig. 7.14).

Vertical mattress sutures

Vertical mattress sutures (Fig. 7.15) are not often used in podiatric surgery, but they do provide a more exact apposition of the wound edges than simple or horizontal mattress sutures. They are used in the avoidance of 'dead space'. However, in some instances the cosmetic result is poor compared with that of other suturing methods.

Method. The needle is inserted approximately twice the distance from the wound edge as used in simple sutures. It is then passed through the tissue to emerge on the other side of the wound a similar distance from the skin edge as the insertion (Fig. 7.15A). The needle is then reinserted into the tissue the same distance from the edge as for a simple suture, passed through the tissue to exit on the far side between the wound edge and the first insertion point, and tied (Fig. 7.15B).

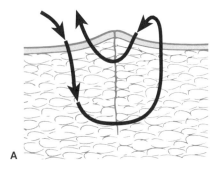
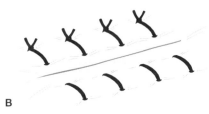

A

B

Figure 7.15 A, B: Vertical mattress suture.

Subcuticular sutures

Subcuticular sutures (Fig. 7.16) are regularly employed in bunion procedures. They may be either absorbable (4/0 Dexon®) or non-absorbable (3/0 Ethilon®) and are usually continuous, horizontally applied intradermal sutures, giving a good cosmetic effect.

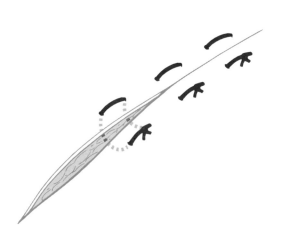

Figure 7.14 Interrupted horizontal mattress suture.

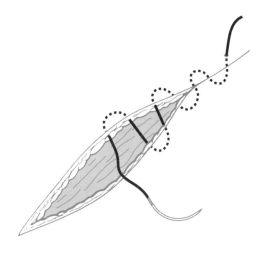

Figure 7.16 Subcuticular suture.

Method. The needle is inserted into the dermis in small equal bites along the length of the wound. The suture is started approximately 1 cm from one end and to one side of the wound with the needle being brought into the wound. The needle is then again taken in the needle holder and a 4 or 5 mm bite of the dermis is taken on the side opposite to the needle entry point. The needle is pulled through the dermis and a further bite is now taken on the other side of the wound with the needle entry exactly opposite the exit point. The bites are continued in this way until reaching the end of the wound. To avoid accidentally crossing the suture and to facilitate everting the skin the surgeon can use forceps on the near side of the wound. Meanwhile on the far side the skin can be everted by the assistant, who follows the suture as the needle is brought to the assistant's side of the wound.

When closing the wound the thread at the entry point is tied in a knot as follows. The thread is wound twice around the forceps, then slid down the forceps blade on to the suture below the tip and tightened (Fig. 7.17). This is repeated but twisting the thread in the opposite direction. The thread is then gently pulled from the opposite end to close the wound and the thread is tied off in the same manner.

Alternatively a small clip, or bead, is crimped to the thread where it enters and leaves the skin.

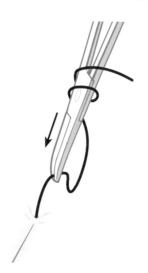

Figure 7.17 Tying a subcuticular suture end knot.

The subcuticular suture can also be closed with a buried knot (Fig. 7.18). The method is similar but the suture is anchored at one end and pulled taut after each bite.

Possible problems with subcuticular sutures

These include the following.

- If a needle with a large curvature is used the bite will be too large and gaping may occur at the centre of each bite because the arc of the needle takes the suture too far from the skin edge.
- When using a non-absorbable suture care must be taken to ensure that it runs freely before tying. If it is not free, remove it.
- If the needle bites overlap or a superficial bite is taken, the suture will not slip through the tissue, but will lock and wrinkle the skin.

Other suture techniques

Modified Donatti and subcuticular apical sutures

When a skin flap is being closed, as in a V plasty, a technique known as a modified Donatti suture (Fig. 7.19) may be used if there is a risk of impaired circulation (note the positioning of the suture). If there is no risk of impaired circulation subcuticular apical suture can be used (Fig. 7.20).

Transfixation suture

Transfixation sutures (Fig. 7.21) are used to close large blood vessels. The needle is inserted through the centre of the vessel and one knot applied (Fig. 7.21A). The thread is then taken around the vessel and tied again (Fig. 7.21B). On occasion the needle may also be inserted into the surrounding tissue and tied to hold the vessel in place. The suture material normally used is a multifilament type such as Dexon®.

Undersewing

If there is continuous bleeding with no obvious source then forceps or diathermy should not be used blindly, as either of these may damage

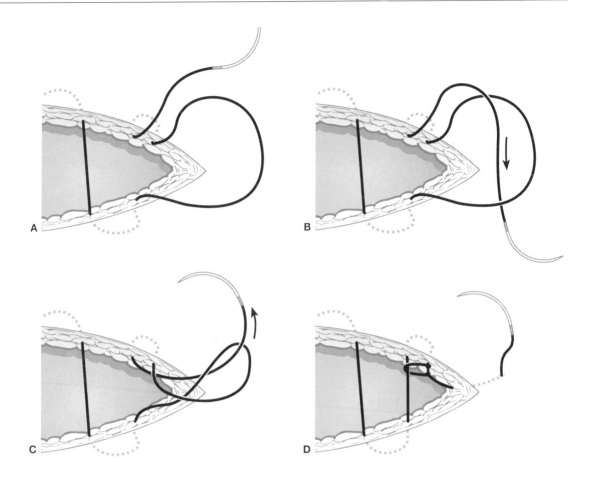

Figure 7.18 A–D: Buried subcuticular knot (end knot).

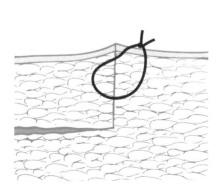

Figure 7.19 Modified Donatti suture.

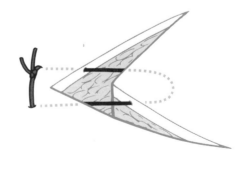

Figure 7.20 Subcuticular apical suture.

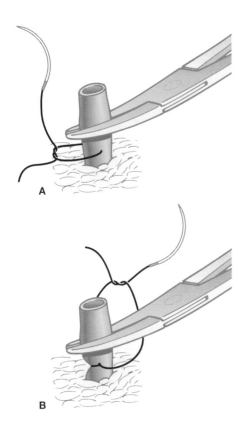

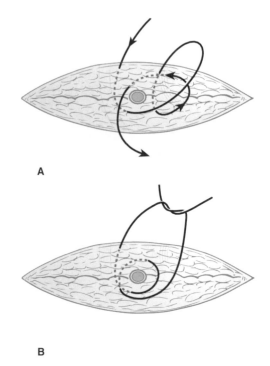

Figure 7.22 A, B: Undersewing.

Figure 7.21 Transfixation suture. A: First knot. B: Second knot.

associated structures. If the bleeding is from a single blood vessel then it is possible that it may have retracted into the tissue; if packing or pressure does not arrest the bleeding then undersewing (Fig. 7.22) may be used with good effect. In this technique, the needle is inserted several times into the area where there is bleeding and then tied off.

Buried knot

A buried knot technique (Fig. 7.23) is often used after the removal of a Morton neuroma, to help avoid 'dead space'. The technique can also be used on shallower wounds, where careful placing of the sutures will bring the tissues together in such a way that final closure can be carried out using only Steristrips®.

An absorbable suture such as Dexon® or Vicryl® is used. The first bite is taken *upwards* through one side of the wound (Fig. 7.23A). The needle is then brought out of the wound and then inserted *downwards* into the opposite side (Fig. 7.23B), then out again and finally tied (Fig. 7.23C, D). Simple hand tying is normally used for the knot.

Suturing a wound with the tissue under tension: undermining

Occasionally during a hammer toe procedure, for example if an ellipse of tissue is removed in the excision of a bursa, the wound then may be too wide to allow the wound edges to be opposed without undue tension (Fig. 7.24). If you simply pull the suture this will often either tear the skin or the too-tight suture, and may cause ischaemic necrosis.

This problem can often be resolved by undermining the wound on either side (Fig. 7.25), although care must be taken not to compromise the blood supply to the flaps. If undermining is not possible it may be better to allow the wound to heal by granulation.

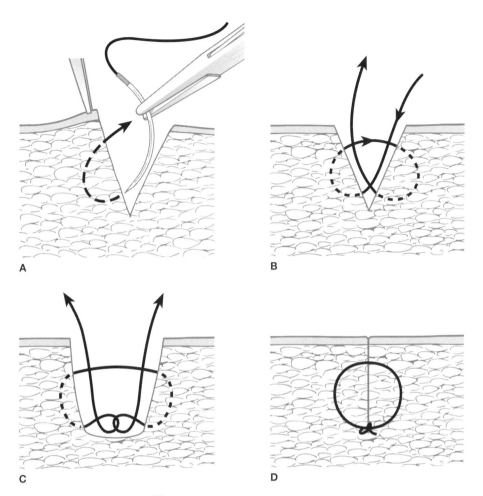

A

B

C

D

Figure 7.23 A–D: Method of tying a buried knot.

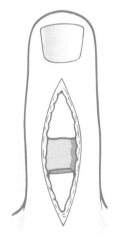

Figure 7.24 Too large an ellipse of tissue removed.

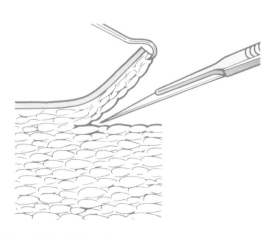

Figure 7.25 Undermining.

Closing a gaping wound

Another method of closing a gaping wound (Fig. 7.26A), or one with sagging edges, is to apply a skin hook at either end and gently pull the wound closed (Fig. 7.26B). The first suture should be placed near the middle of the wound, and subsequent sutures then bisect the gap. This should avoid a possible 'dog ear'.

Dog ear

When wound edges are incorrectly aligned then 'dog ears' can be created (Fig. 7.27A). Small ears can be flattened out by simply reducing the space between the sutures. With larger dog ears this may not be possible in which case the ear is pulled gently with a skin hook (Fig. 7.27B) and the surplus skin excised (Fig. 7.27C).

SKIN BIOPSY, EXCISION BIOPSY

When removing a section of tissue for excision biopsy the lesion should be completely removed. An elliptical incision is made, the length of the ellipse being four times its width. The margin of skin around the lesion will depend on the suspected diagnosis. For benign

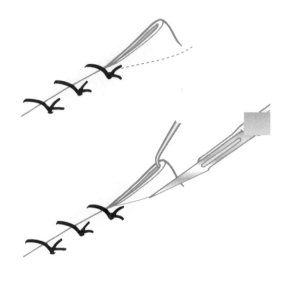

Figure 7.27   A–C: Removing a dog ear.

lesions a full thickness ellipse of skin is removed with a minimum of 1 to 2 mm margin of normal skin either side of the lesion. If a basal cell carcinoma is suspected, however, a clearance of at least 3 mm must be allowed, and around a squamous cell carcinoma a clearance of 5 mm.

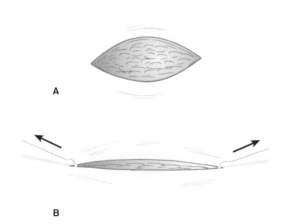

A

B

Figure 7.26   A, B: Using skin hooks to help in wound closure.

TIP: Place a suture at one end of the tissue sample to orientate the sample for the pathologist (Fig. 7.28). Don't forget to mention on the pathology request form whether the suture is attached to the proximal or the distal edge of the sample.

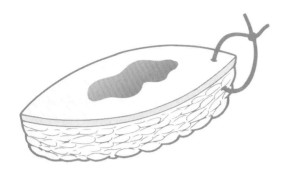

Figure 7.28 Suture in place to orientate a skin sample.

REMOVING SUTURES

Sutures are normally removed 14 days after foot surgery, although patients on steroids or with impaired healing should have the sutures left in position for a further 2 to 4 days. If sutures are left in place for too long this can lead to infection, incorporation of the suture by epithelialization, scarring and pain. If the suture has to be removed early because of infection the wound should not be resutured but supported by Steristrips®. Non-absorbable subcuticular sutures may be left in for longer periods if the wound edges require support, although there will be the possibility of scarring or sinus formation at the entry and exit points.

It is important to inspect the wound to confirm that healing has occurred before removing any suture.

> **TIP:** Check the operative notes before removing the sutures, especially when subcuticular sutures are used. It may seem obvious, but absorbable subcuticular sutures are not removed (some people have tried); only the end knots are cut.

The suture may be cut with a no. 11 or 15 blade, or a disposable stitch cutter. Although there is no set order for removing sutures from a wound it is better to remove the sutures from different parts of a long wound to confirm that the wound has healed before removing all of them.

Removing a simple suture

To remove a simple interrupted suture, first one end of the suture is picked up with forceps to lift it off the skin. The suture is then cut flush to the skin and removed. Be careful not to pull on the wound edges (Fig. 7.29A).

Removing a mattress suture

Here the loop opposite the knot is lifted with the forceps and both stems of the loop are cut (Fig. 7.29B). The suture is then removed by pulling on the knot.

Removing a non-absorbable subcuticular suture

One end of the suture is first lifted and cut flush with the skin. The other end is held by artery forceps and gently pulled. At the same time the edges of the wound are protected by moderate pressure from the fingers of your other hand. The pull is increased until the suture starts to slide. As it is pulled through the skin, move your fingers along

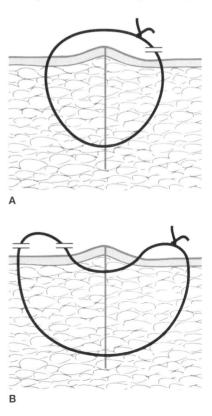

Figure 7.29 Where to cut sutures for removal. A: Simple interrupted sutures. B: Vertical mattress sutures.

slightly behind it. If the suture snags and breaks it may be better to leave it in place than to dig into the wound. In most instances the end of the suture will work its way out spontaneously, at which point it can easily be removed.

Removing Steristrips®

If Steristrips® have been used in conjunction with a subcuticular suture they should be removed at the same time. The easiest way to do this is to use non-toothed forceps. Lift one end of the strip towards the wound. Then lift the other end, also towards the wound. When both ends are together then lift the strip perpendicularly and along the line of the wound. (If the strip is lifted from one side only and pulled this may cause one edge of the wound to lift.)

8

Instruments used in podiatry

As surgical assistant you will be expected to be familiar with *all* of the instruments that will be used during podiatric surgery. At first glance there appear to be too many to remember. Don't worry though—you will not be expected to remember the names of all of them, at least not at first. In any case it is not unusual for the same instrument to be called by another name at a different hospital. Fortunately for the new assistant there are only a limited number of instruments that are regularly used in podiatric surgery and these are displayed later in this chapter.

CLEANING INSTRUMENTS

In the majority of cases the instruments used in the podiatry surgical unit will arrive in prepacked containers from the hospital sterilization department or surgical suppliers. However, there will undoubtedly be occasions when you will have to clean and sterilize the instruments before the next operation.

> **TIP:** The operative staff and the patient place their trust and welfare in your care during this important process.

Something that you may not realize is that even though an instrument has gone through an autoclave it may *not* be sterile. Irrespective of the autoclaving system employed the total sterilization of an instrument cannot be guaranteed if there are any fragments of bone or dried blood attached to it. Any instrument found in this condition cannot be used until it has been cleaned again and resterilized.

TIP: Dried blood is a breeding place for bacteria, no matter where it is.

Any blood that is on an instrument in the autoclave will dry on to the instrument, effectively becoming part of it. This makes it very difficult if not impossible to remove totally. If this is the case that instrument has to be discarded.

TIP: Take care when cleaning some power tools as you may not be able to submerse them totally in any form of cleaning fluid.

Before placing instruments in the autoclave you must scrub all instruments that are suitable for this. Take particular care when cleaning toothed or grooved instruments such as haemostats and needle holders.

TIP: Scissor-like instruments are by far the most difficult to clean as blood can accumulate between the blades and around the screw.

Ideally instruments should be placed in an ultrasonic cleaner for at least 3 minutes before scrubbing. After using this cleaner the instruments must then be washed in distilled water to remove the cleaning fluid before placing them in the autoclave. Failure to do so can lead to discoloration or pitting.

TIP: Some air-driven instruments should not be placed in an ultrasonic cleaner as the cleaner may cause damage to the bearings in the handpiece. Read the manufacturer's instructions before cleaning.

Considerations when cleaning and using instruments

Always:

- use the instrument only for the purpose that it was designed for
- check the manufacturer's instructions before using and before cleaning instruments, particularly power-driven instruments; lubricate after cleaning only if required (some air-driven handpieces should never be lubricated because of the risk of explosion if the propellant gas mixes with the lubricant)
- handle instruments gently; don't knock them together
- check all instruments for damage after use
- dismantle scissor-like instruments if necessary, then clean them in cold water as soon as possible after use, removing all blood, bone and tissue fragments from their serrations, joints and ratchets
- if using a detergent in an ultrasonic cleaner ensure it is of the recommended strength
- after cleaning ensure that all instruments are thoroughly dried before being stored
- when packing instruments in instrument packs, ensure that the heavier ones are at the bottom of the pack.

Never:

- leave dirty instruments to dry
- use abrasives on instruments
- use general purpose lubricants or oils; use only water-soluble lubricants
- use damaged instruments
- store damp instruments
- leave instruments soaking longer than required in chemical cleaning agents
- place instruments with contaminants on them in an autoclave.

BASIC INSTRUMENT PACK

Each hospital or podiatric department will have its own version of the basic podiatric surgical pack. Therefore the following should be taken only *as an example* of the basic arthroplasty pack used for most podiatric surgical procedures, with other instruments being added as required.

Basic arthroplasty pack

The basic pack for arthroplasty is illustrated in Figure 8.1. It comprises the following instruments:

- no. 3 scalpel handle   (2)
- Kilner needle holder   (2)
- towel clamps   (5)
- Allis tissue forceps   (1)
- Mayo safety pin forceps holder   (1)
- haemostat curved   (2)
- haemostat straight   (3)
- toothed dissecting forceps   (1)
- Stamm bone cutter   (1)
- bone rongeur   (1)

- Gillies skin hook   (2)
- Bell (bone) rasp   (1)
- Kilner retractor   (2)
- bone-holding forceps   (1)
- Mayo curved scissors   (1)
- Metzenbaum straight scissors   (1)

ADDITIONAL INSTRUMENTS FOR OTHER PROCEDURES

The additional instruments required for particular procedures will depend greatly on the particular requirements of the individual podiatrist. Some podiatrists, for example, prefer to use a mallet and osteotome as opposed to power equipment when reducing a simple metatarsal exostosis.

Some surgical procedures that may require additional instruments include the following.

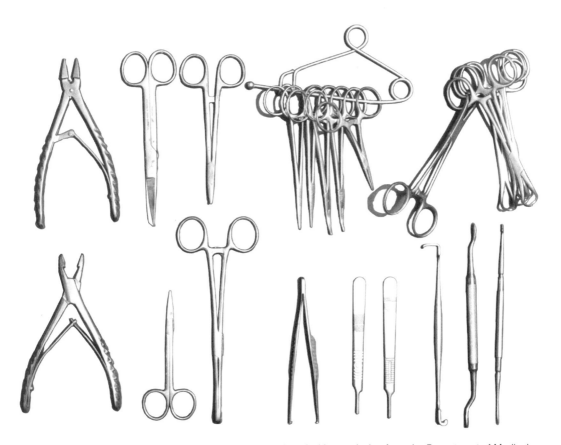

Figure 8.1 Basic arthroplasty pack (without extras). (Reproduced with permission from the Department of Medical Illustration, Ipswich Hospital NHS Trust, Ipswich, UK.)

Keller's arthroplasty

This operation is illustrated in Figure 8.2.

Additional instruments that are required for the operation include the following:

- power saw, with blades   (1)
- Langenbeck retractor   (1)
- flat metatarsal retractor   (1)
- Hohmann bone elevator (Fig. 8.3)   (2)
- saw blades   (as required)

Silver's bunionectomy

This requires the same additional instruments as for the Keller's arthroplasty. However, some podiatrists may prefer to use a mallet and osteotome in place of the powered saw. The operation is shown in Figure 8.4.

Austin osteotomy

This is sometimes known as a chevron osteotomy. In this procedure the metatarsal head is cut

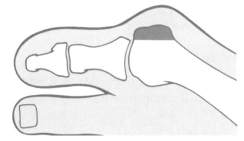

Figure 8.4 Silver's bunionectomy. The shaded area represents where the bone will be removed.

at a 60° angle. Then the head is moved laterally and fixed into position with a K wire. The operation is shown in Figure 8.5.

Additional instruments required are as follows:

- power saw, with 3 blades   (1)
- K wires (size as required)
- power K-wire driver   (1)
- Langenbeck retractor   (2)
- K-wire-bending tool (may be an Adson
  suction tube (Fig. 8.6) or similar)
- wire-cutting forceps   (1)
- flat metatarsal retractor   (1)
- double-ended, flat/round probe   (1)

As a precaution it may be advisable to have a reel of suturing wire, in the (rare) event that the

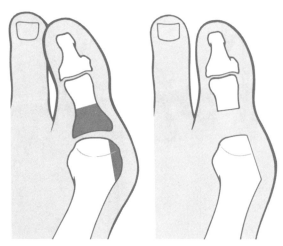

Figure 8.2 Keller's arthroplasty. A: Before the operation. The shaded areas represent where the bone will be removed. B: After the operation.

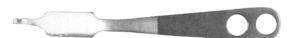

Figure 8.3 Hohmann bone elevator.

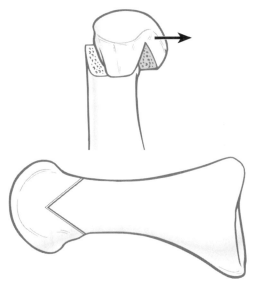

Figure 8.5 Austin osteotomy.

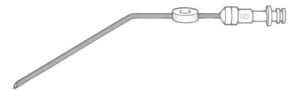

Figure 8.6 Adson suction tube.

metatarsal head fractures as it is being repositioned.

Excision of Morton's neuroma

For this operation the following are needed:

- Weitlander retractor (1)
- Metzenbaum scissors (delicate)
  curved or flat (1)

Nail avulsion (partial/total)

See Chapter 5 and Figure 5.1.

SCALPEL BLADES

The different types and sizes of scalpel blades required are shown in Figure 8.7.

OTHER MISCELLANEOUS INSTRUMENTS

A variety of other instruments are used during podiatric surgery. These are illustrated in Figure 8.8. (See also Figs 2.3, p. 24; 2.11, p. 33; 4.3, p. 54; 4.4, p. 55; 4.7, p. 56; 4.14, p. 59; 4.16, p. 60; 5.4, p. 71; 5.7 and 5.8, p. 73; 5.10, p. 76; 7.12, p. 88.)

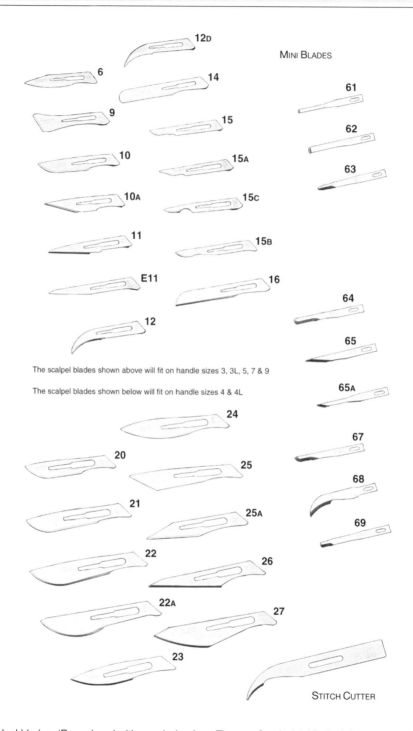

Figure 8.7 Scalpel blades. (Reproduced with permission from Timesco Surgical & Medical, London, UK.)

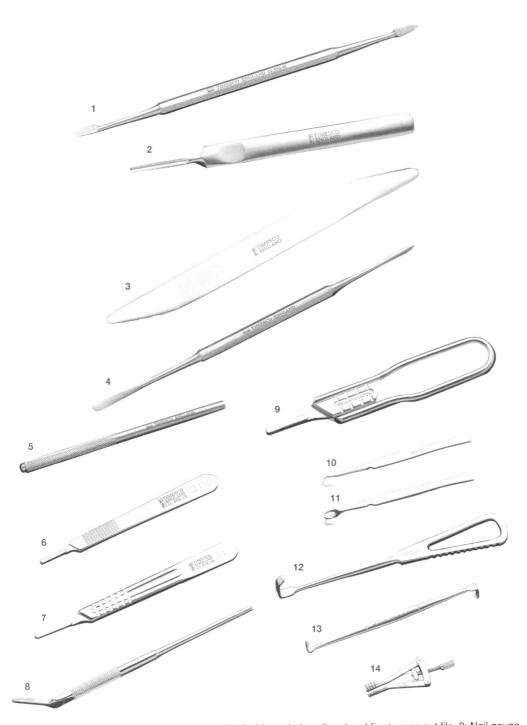

Figure 8.8   Instruments used in podiatry. 1: A 15 cm (6") double-ended medium head fine/coarse cut file. 2: Nail gouge. 3: Mackay double-ended elevator. 4: Double-ended shallow curved round/point elevator. 5: Beaver (chuck) handle. 6: No. 3 scalpel handle. 7: No. 4 scalpel handle. 8: Round no. 3 angled scalpel handle. 9: No. 4 folding alloy scalpel handle. 10: Single hook retractor (sharp). 11: Double hook retractor (sharp). 12: Langenbeck retractor. 13: T retractor, double-ended blunt. 14: Alm skin self-retraining retractor.

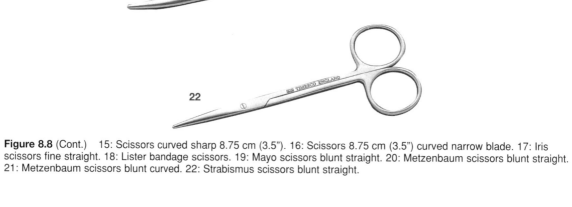

Figure 8.8 (Cont.)   15: Scissors curved sharp 8.75 cm (3.5"). 16: Scissors 8.75 cm (3.5") curved narrow blade. 17: Iris scissors fine straight. 18: Lister bandage scissors. 19: Mayo scissors blunt straight. 20: Metzenbaum scissors blunt straight. 21: Metzenbaum scissors blunt curved. 22: Strabismus scissors blunt straight.

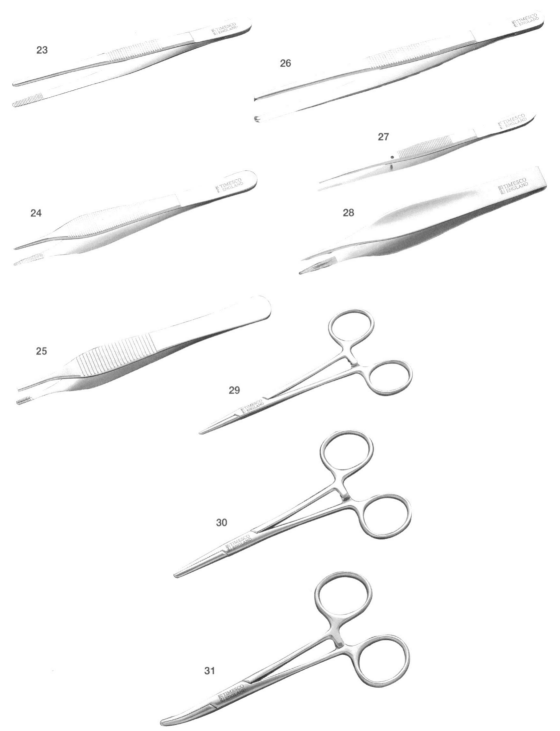

Figure 8.8 (Cont.)   23: Broad serrated end forceps. 24: Adson dissecting forceps serrated. 25: Adson Brown forceps 9 × 9 teeth. 26: Broad forceps 1 × 2 teeth. 27: Iris forceps serrated fine point. 28: Splinter forceps. 29: Halstead mosquito forceps. 30: Spencer Wells forceps. 31: Spencer Wells curved forceps.

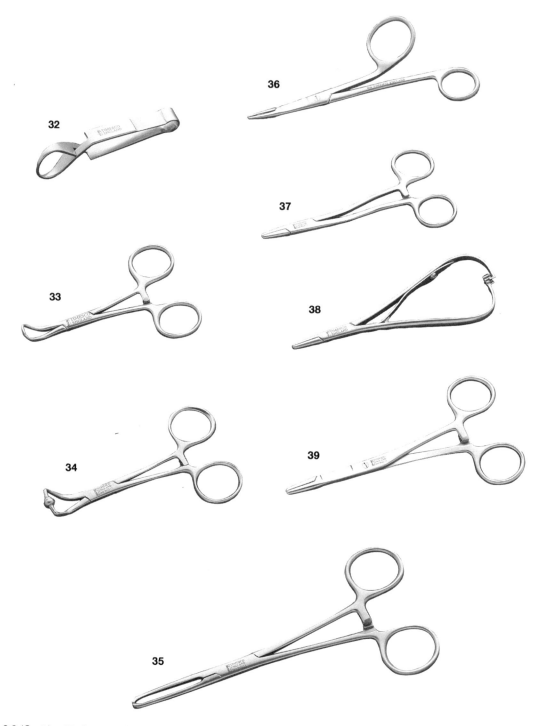

Figure 8.8 (Cont.)   32: Cross-action towel clip. 33: Bachaus towel forceps. 34: Bachaus atraumatic ball-and-socket towel forceps. 35: Allis tissue forceps. 36: Gillies right-hand scissors and needle holder. 37: Kilner needle holder. 38: Mathieu needle holder. 39: Olsen needle holder.

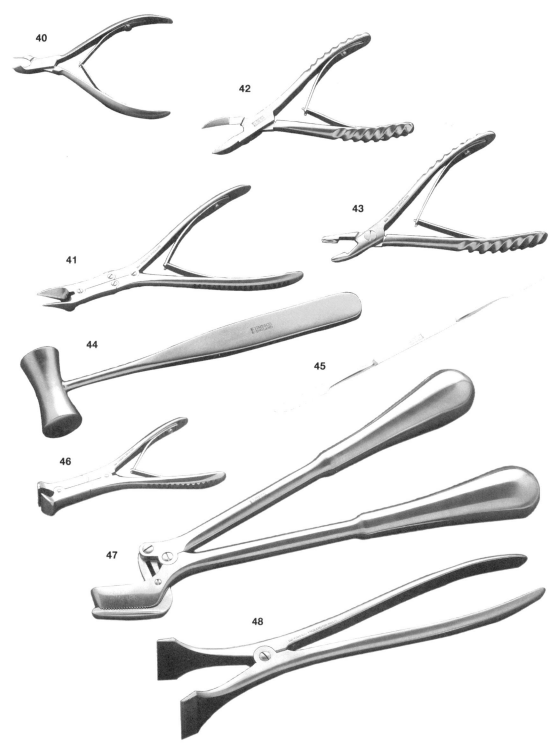

Figure 8.8 (Cont.)   40: Cuticle and tissue cutter. 41: Angled bone-cutting forceps. 42: Stamm bone-cutting forceps. 43: Bone rongeur. 44: Surgical mallet. 45: MacDonald double-ended dissector. 46: Wire-cutting forceps. 47: Stille serrated plaster shears. 48: Henning plaster spreader.

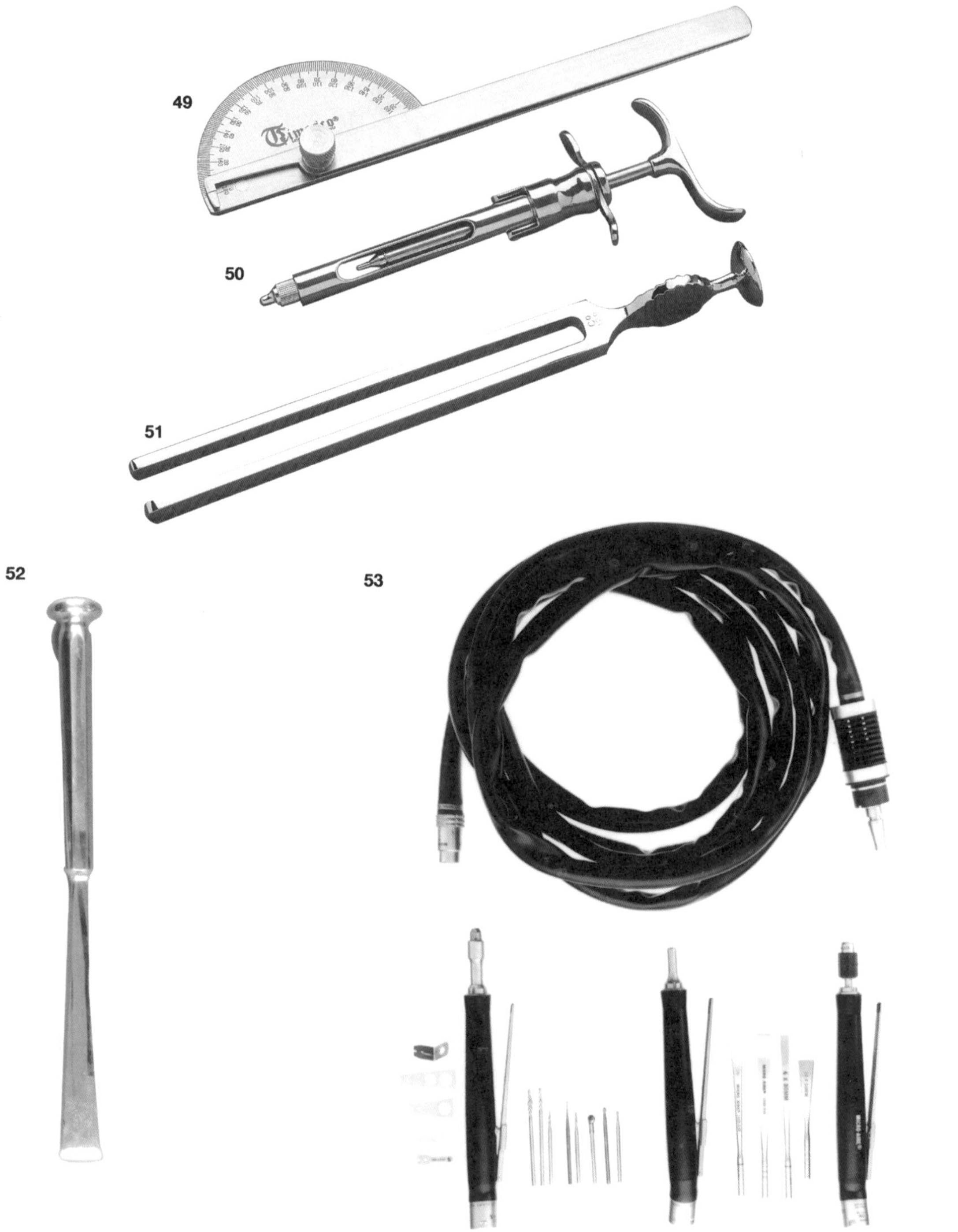

Figure 8.8 (Cont.) 49: Goniometer. 50: Cartridge syringe. 51: Tuning fork. 52: Osteotome. 53: Micro Aire drill and K-wire driver. (52 & 53 reproduced with permission from the Department of Medical Illustration, Ipswich Hospital NHS Trust, Ipswich, UK. Other photos reproduced with permission from Timesco Surgical & Medical, London, UK.)

9

Clinical emergencies

Serious clinical medical emergencies are fortunately rare although in your work as a podiatric surgical assistant you may encounter a wide range of minor accidents and emergencies. As a podiatric surgical assistant you should be familiar with all of the emergency facilities in your department. You should also be proficient in at least basic life support (BLS).

If an emergency occurs, you must:

1. cease any podiatric procedure
2. call for assistance
3. remain with the patient to monitor and provide assistance or administer appropriate therapy
4. remain calm
5. if required carry out the emergency action plan, either BLS or cardiopulmonary resuscitation (CPR), as appropriate; remember the ABC—**A**irway, **B**reathing, **C**irculation.

BASIC LIFE SUPPORT

The term 'basic life support' is used to imply that the rescuer has no equipment of any kind. If any form of mouth ventilation or face mask is used—for example a Laerdal pocket mask or Guedel airway—the procedure is termed 'basic life support with airway adjunct'.

Laerdal pocket mask

This is a piece of equipment ideally suited for use in podiatry clinics. The mask is carried in a collapsed state. It has a one-way valve and a securing head strap (Fig. 9.1A). The mask is placed in position and held securely by the rescuer with two hands; the rescuer simultaneously produces a jaw-thrust. This enables ventilation to be given effectively without direct mouth-to-mouth contact. It also avoids the patient's exhaled air being inhaled by the rescuer (Fig. 9.1B). If oxygen is available it can be administered through the nipple on the Laerdal mask.

Guedel airway

A Guedel airway (Fig. 9.2A) is inserted with its tip pointing towards the roof of the mouth. It is then rotated through 180° to advance it fully into position (Fig. 9.2B).

Sequence of actions in BLS

The procedure is as follows (Fig. 9.3).

1. Ensure that both you and the patient are safe.
2. Check for responsiveness by gently shaking the patient's shoulders and asking loudly: 'Are you all right?'.
3. If the patient responds then he or she can be left in the position found (if in no further danger). Check the person's condition and obtain help if required. Whilst waiting for help, reassess the patient's condition regularly.

If the patient does not respond:

1. Shout for help.
2. After ensuring there is no obstruction in the patient's mouth, open the airway by tilting the head and lifting the chin (Fig. 9.4). The

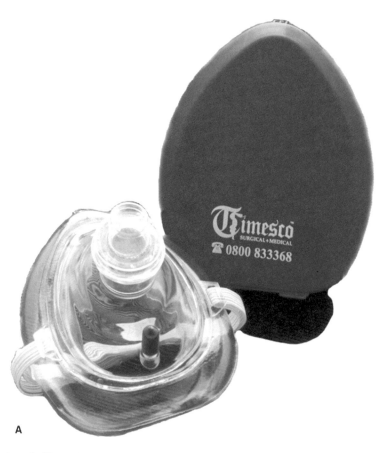

A

Figure 9.1 A: Pocket mask. (Reproduced with permission from Timesco Surgical & Medical, London, UK.)

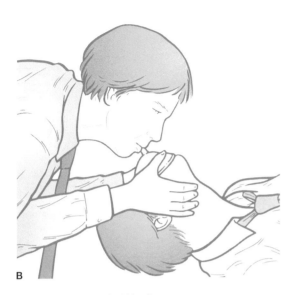

Figure 9.1   B: Mask held in place.

procedure is as follows. First, place your hand on the patient's forehead and gently tilt the head back keeping your thumb and index finger free to close the nose if rescue breathing is required. Keeping your fingertips under the point of the patient's chin, lift the chin to open the airway.

3. Keeping the airway open, look, listen and feel for any breathing (listen at the patient's mouth for sounds of breathing, and feel for air on your cheek). You should look, listen and feel for up to 10 seconds before deciding whether the person is breathing.

4. If the person is breathing:

   4.1 place the patient in the recovery position (Fig. 9.5)

   4.2 check for continued breathing

   4.3 send someone for assistance.

Even though the patient continues breathing, it is still important to maintain a good airway and to ensure that the tongue does not fall back and cause an obstruction. The recovery position allows the tongue to fall forward, keeping the airway clear. It will also reduce the risk of

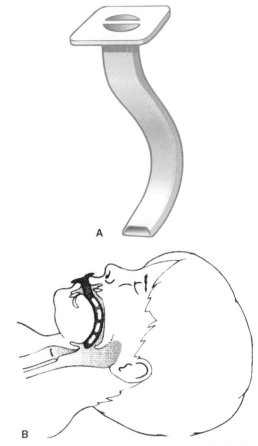

Figure 9.2   A, B: Guedel airway. (Part B reproduced with permission from Chellel A (ed.) 2000 Resuscitation: A guide for nurses. Churchill Livingstone, Edinburgh, p. 130.)

inhalation of gastric contents if the patient vomits.

Sequence for placing a patient into the recovery position

1. Kneel beside the patient, and straighten both of the person's legs.

2. Tuck the patient's hand that is nearest to you, with the arm straight and palm uppermost, well under the person's buttock.

3. With one hand, bring the person's far arm across the chest and hold the back of the person's hand against the nearest cheek.

4. With your other hand, grasp the person's far leg just above the knee and pull it up, but keeping the foot on the ground.

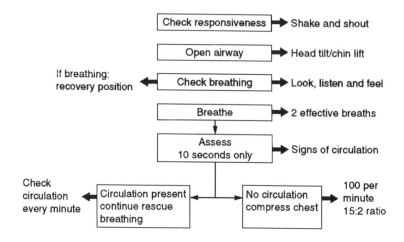

Figure 9.3 flow chart content:

Check responsiveness → Shake and shout

Open airway → Head tilt/chin lift

If breathing: recovery position ← Check breathing → Look, listen and feel

Breathe → 2 effective breaths

Assess 10 seconds only → Signs of circulation

Check circulation every minute ← Circulation present continue rescue breathing → No circulation compress chest → 100 per minute 15:2 ratio

Send or go for help as soon as possible according to guidelines

Figure 9.3 Basic life support. 1. Check responsiveness: shake and shout. If unresponsive, shout for help. 2. Open airway: head tilt, chin lift. 3. Check breathing: look, listen, feel (up to 10 s). If breathing present, place in recovery position. 4. If no breathing present, give two effective breaths. 5. Assess circulation: movement, pulse (no more than 10 s). 6a. If circulation is present, continue rescue breathing; check circulation every minute. 6b. If no circulation, compress the chest: 100/min, 15 : 2 ratio. (Reproduced with permission from Chellel A (ed.) 2000 Resuscitation: A guide for nurses. Churchill Livingstone, Edinburgh, p. 68.)

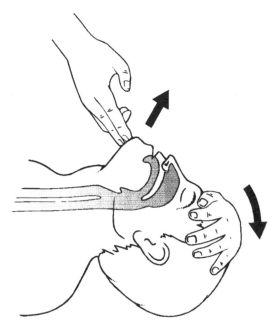

Figure 9.4 Head tilt and chin lift manoeuvre. (Reproduced with permission from Chellel A (ed.) 2000 Resuscitation: A guide for nurses. Churchill Livingstone, Edinburgh, p. 128.)

5. Keeping the person's hand pressed against the cheek, pull on the leg to roll the patient towards you on to one side.

6. Adjust the upper leg so that both the hip and knee are bent at right angles.
7. Move the person's lower arm so that the patient is lying on it.
8. Tilt the head back to ensure that the airway remains open.
9. Adjust the hand under the cheek, to keep the head tilted (Fig. 9.5).
10. Check the breathing.

If the patient is not breathing:

1. Send someone for help.
2. Turn the patient on to their back.

Sequence for turning a patient on to their back

1. Kneel by the patient's side and place the arm nearest to you above the person's head.
2. Turn the head to face away from you.
3. Grasp the patient's far shoulder with one hand and the hip with the other.
4. With a steady but firm pull roll the patient against your thighs.
5. Lower the person gently to the ground on to the back, supporting the head as you do so.

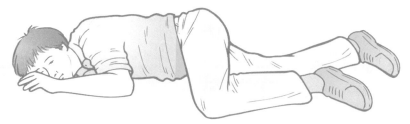

Figure 9.5 Recovery position.

Sequence for rescue breathing

1. When the patient is lying on the back remove any visible obstructions from the patient's mouth (well-fitting dentures should be left in place).
2. Give two effective breaths, each of which should make the chest rise and fall.
3. Maintain the head tilt and chin lift.
4. Pinch the soft part of the patient's nose closed with the thumb and index finger of your hand that is on the patient's forehead.
5. Open the patient's mouth a little, maintaining the chin lift.
6. Take a breath and place your lips around the patient's mouth, making sure that you have a good seal.
7. Blow steadily into the patient's mouth for about 1.5 to 2 seconds, watching for the chest to rise.

> **TIP:** If you breathe into the patient in the form of a hard puff, you may cause the patient to vomit, as your breath would most probably enter the patient's stomach and not the lungs.

8. Whilst maintaining head tilt and chin lift, take your mouth away from the patient and watch for the chest to fall as the air comes out.
9. Take another breath and repeat the sequence. *Give two effective rescue breaths in all.*

Assessing the circulation and cardiopulmonary resuscitation

Assess the circulation as follows:

1. Look for any movement.
2. Check the carotid pulse. Take no more than 10 seconds to do this.

If you can detect signs of circulation within 10 seconds, continue rescue breathing until the patient starts breathing unaided. If the patient breathes unaided but remains unconscious, place the person in the recovery position.

If there is no sign of returned circulation then start chest compression, as follows.

First, locate the lower half of the sternum (breastbone) (Fig. 9.6A).

Use your index and middle fingers to identify the lower rib margins. Then keeping your fingers together, slide them upwards towards the point where the ribs join the sternum. With your middle finger on this point, place your index finger on the sternum next to it.

Now slide the heel of your other hand down the sternum until it is next to your index finger. This hand should now be over the middle of the lower half of the sternum. Place the heel of the hand there and then place the other hand on top. Interlock and then lift the fingers so as to avoid applying pressure to the ribs (Fig. 9.6B).

Position yourself vertically above the patient's chest and then *with your arms straight* press down on the sternum to depress it 2.5–5 cm (or 1–2") (Fig. 9.6C).

Release the pressure, then repeat. The rate is about 100 compressions a minute (approximately two compressions a second) (Fig. 9.6D).

> **TIP:** Remember that if the patient is on a bed that has a 'springy mattress', a wooden bed board should be used under the person, or the patient may have to be removed from the bed and placed on the floor.

Combine the rescue breathing and compressions as follows. *After 15 compressions tilt the head, lift the chin and give two effective breaths.* Then

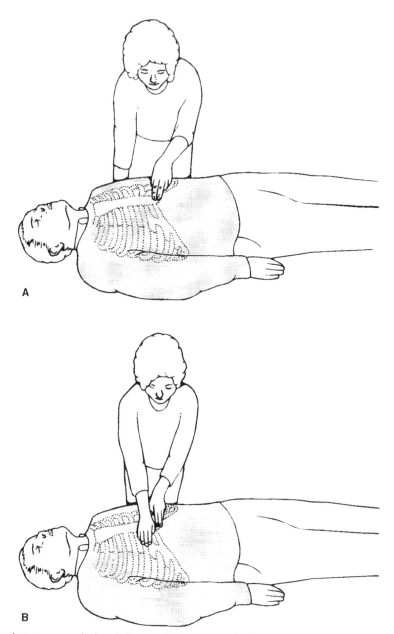

Figure 9.6 Cardiopulmonary resuscitation. A: Lower middle sternum. B, C: Heel of one hand over other.

return your hands to the sternum and give a further 15 compressions. *Continue with the compressions and breaths in a 15 : 2 ratio.*

You should continue resuscitation until:

- the patient shows signs of life
- qualified help arrives
- you become exhausted.

CLINICAL EMERGENCIES

Cardiac arrest

A patient is considered to have suffered a cardiac arrest if the person is both unconscious and has no pulse—in other words where there is an absence of a major pulse (i.e. carotid).

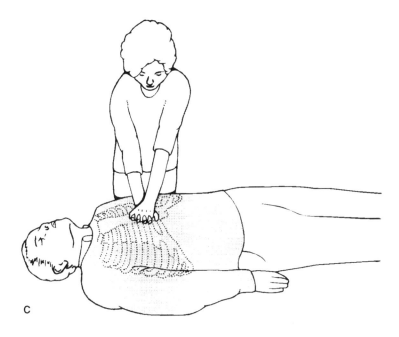

C

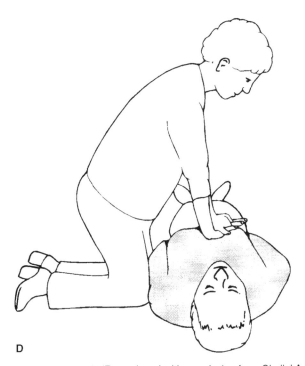

D

Figure 9.6 (Cont.)   D: Compress 2.5–5 cm (1–2"). (Reproduced with permission from Chellel A (ed.) 2000 Resuscitation: A guide for nurses. Churchill Livingstone, Edinburgh, pp. 76–77.)

> **TIP:** Signs such as pupil size, cyanosis or pallor are unreliable. Information such as the time of the collapse, age, medical history, current medication, whether there was chest pain before or after collapse, time CPR commenced will be of importance to the hospital emergency staff.

Management

1. Call for assistance. If in hospital call for the arrest team (don't forget to tell them where you are).

2. Commence BLS.

3. If the cause of the arrest was *not* witnessed remember the basic ABC: **A**irway, **B**reathing, **C**irculation.

4. If you *witness* the collapse then give a precordial thump, check the pulse if it is absent, and begin BLS with 15–30 compressions *before* ventilation; the order in this case is CAB: **C**irculation, **A**irway, **B**reathing. The rationale of this approach is that *at the moment of collapse in a patient with a sudden ventricular fibrillation (VF) the lungs and arterial blood are still well oxygenated; therefore the most urgent treatment is to restore the circulation— by chest compressions.*

Resuscitation should be continued until the ambulance or crash team arrive. The podiatrist will have been trained in advanced cardiac life support (see below) so will be able to use the defibrillator if one is available.

Advanced treatment (Fig. 9.7)

The treatment in this case, unless you have had special training, will be carried out by the podiatrist or hospital emergency staff. It consists of maintaining an airway, and administering high-flow oxygen and epinephrine. (The latter should be given in small aliquots, e.g. 0.1 mg every 2–3 minutes intravenously, or intramuscularly if the veins have collapsed.) You should also be prepared to carry out CPR until the hospital emergency team arrive.

Anaphylaxis

Anaphylaxis can be described as a rapidly occurring hypersensitivity reaction with a possibly fatal response to a drug. The most probable cause seen in podiatry will be the administration of a local anaesthetic.

The reaction consists of respiratory distress, cyanosis accompanied by peripheral circulatory collapse, hypotension and shock. In a severe reaction the patient will rapidly become unconscious. You should commence BLS.

Allergic reactions to drugs can vary from mild to severe, even fatal, reactions. An indication of the severity of the reaction is the time that has elapsed between the administration of the drug and the reaction. If the reaction occurs less than 1 hour after receipt of the drug it is potentially life threatening. Reactions that occur more than 1 hour later are generally benign.

Angina (chest pain)

The pain of angina is caused by a reduction in the blood supply to the heart. This generally does no harm to the heart providing it does not progress to a severe complication such as myocardial infarction (MI).

Patients who suffer from angina normally carry with them some form of medication, possibly glyceryl trinitrate as tablets or in the form of a spray. An attack may be brought on by overexertion or emotional stress. The pain of angina pectoris is typically substernal and often radiates to the left shoulder and arm, or occasionally to the right shoulder and arm or the left side of the neck and jaw.

A sharp stabbing pain is not typical of angina. The patients normally describe angina pain as a dull squeezing or tightening of the chest. Patients who have previously had attacks will normally recognize the signs and will ask for their medication. The patient should be allowed to sit up, and a tablet should be placed under the tongue (i.e. sublingually). This usually provides relief in under 5 minutes. Oxygen may also be given. The patient should then be transferred to the hospital.

> **TIP:** If the patient's medication does not relieve the pain then the possibility of an acute myocardial infarction must be considered.

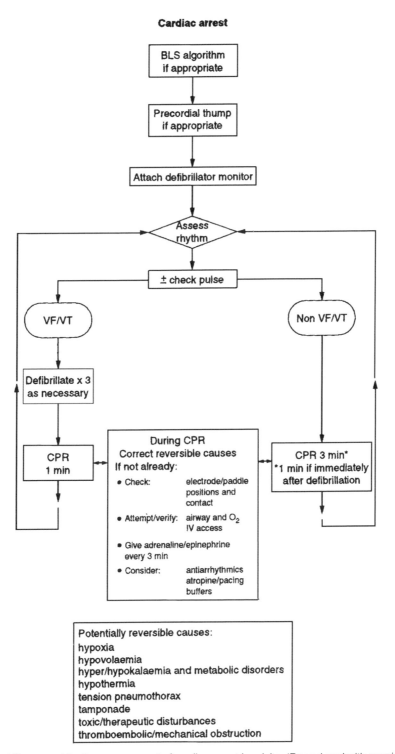

Cardiac arrest

BLS algorithm
if appropriate

Precordial thump
if appropriate

Attach defibrillator monitor

Assess
rhythm

± check pulse

VF/VT

Non VF/VT

Defibrillate x 3
as necessary

CPR
1 min

During CPR
Correct reversible causes
If not already:

• Check: electrode/paddle
positions and
contact

• Attempt/verify: airway and O_2
IV access

• Give adrenaline/epinephrine
every 3 min

• Consider: antiarrhythmics
atropine/pacing
buffers

CPR 3 min*
*1 min if immediately
after defibrillation

Potentially reversible causes:
hypoxia
hypovolaemia
hyper/hypokalaemia and metabolic disorders
hypothermia
tension pneumothorax
tamponade
toxic/therapeutic disturbances
thromboembolic/mechanical obstruction

Figure 9.7 Advanced life support for the management of cardiac arrest in adults. (Reproduced with permission from Chellel A (ed.) 2000 Resuscitation: A guide for nurses. Churchill Livingstone, Edinburgh, p. 83.)

Acute myocardial infarction (MI)

The presentation of a myocardial infarction is normally straightforward. The pain may well be similar to that of angina. *The pain is never sharp*, nor does it start instantaneously. It is often described as squeezing, an ache, tightness or a weight on the chest. Patients who have angina will notice that the pain is more intense in nature and occurs at rest, and is not relieved by their normal medication. The pain of an infarct is often, but not inevitably, accompanied by sweating and nausea. *The patient must be transferred to the hospital.* The patient may also be given an aspirin (to chew) and oxygen if available.

Epilepsy

There are various forms and degrees of epileptic attack. A mild attack may comprise a few moments of inattention and memory loss; it is known as a 'petit mal' and is *not* associated with convulsive movements. This form of attack resembles a faint and should be treated as such.

The more serious attack is known as a 'grand mal'. The grand mal seizure is often preceded by an aura that warns the patient that an attack is about to begin. This can be in the form of a sensation of nausea, odour or a visual flash, after which the patient loses consciousness and falls to the floor. The patient may now lie still in a stiff position for some time, although normally for only a few seconds, during which time the neck becomes congested and cyanosed. This will then be followed by severe, rhythmic synchronous movements of the body. The breathing may become noisy (breathing through a clenched jaw). At this time sphincter control is often lost, and on occasions the tongue may be bitten. This is followed by a period of sleep, when the muscles become relaxed; this phase can last a number of hours.

If the patient suffers a grand mal seizure, you should prevent the patient from inflicting injury to themselves and keep the airway clear. During a spasm protect the patient by gentle restraint but *do not forcibly restrict the person's movements*. If the opportunity arises, remove any spectacles or false teeth and try to put a rolled handkerchief or padded tongue depressor between the patient's jaws, but do *not* try to prise open the mouth. If the patient is unconscious place the person in the recovery position.

Do not leave the patient until the person has made a full recovery. The patient may act in a strange way and wander about without realizing it (postepileptic automatism). You must ask the patient to see his or her doctor. The patient should be allowed to leave the department only in the company of a responsible adult.

> **TIP:** If the attack occurs in the podiatry department it is probably advisable to have the patient transferred to medical care within the hospital as soon as possible.

Hysterical fits

These may be the result of an emotional upset or mental stress. The attack may well simulate an epileptic fit, but it will be more dramatic. The patient may be staging the fit to appeal to the audience. The fit can vary from a shout or scream, or crying to a dramatic rolling on the ground, but with the patient taking care not to inflict self-injury, with arms flying, possibly crying out and pulling the hair. All you can do in a case like this is to stop any podiatric treatment. Reassure the patient gently but firmly. The patient should be kept under observation until sufficiently recovered, and then allowed to leave in the care of a responsible adult.

> **TIP:** Ensure that you enter into the patient's notes any treatment prior to the hysterical fit, as well as a description of the fit. Include especially any medication or injection that may have been administered to the patient because the patient may later claim that the fit was a direct result of the administered drug.

Diabetic comas (insulin and diabetic)

Insulin coma (insulin shock)

This is the most likely type to be encountered during your work as a podiatry assistant. The patient will be hypoglycaemic having failed to eat but *will have taken insulin*.

TIP: Consider the possibility that the patient may have been incorrectly advised (often by a friend) that nothing should be eaten prior to the operation. If this is to be carried out under a local anaesthetic there is normally no dietary restriction.

The patient may appear mentally dulled, drowsy, sometimes abnormally aggressive, or confused and may act as if drunk. Classically the patient is pale with profuse sweating but with a cold skin temperature, a rapid pulse and shallow breathing—*the breath is odourless*. The person may faint or become unconscious. It should be remembered that if a patient has been on insulin treatment for some time the warning symptoms of an impending coma may well become less evident.

TIP: Have a glucose drink on hand in the department.

The treatment is to administer a sugar-containing drink or give the patient lumps of sugar. If there is a dramatic improvement then the problem was one of excess insulin. If there is no improvement it is possible that the patient is experiencing a *diabetic coma*. If the person faints or loses consciousness then place in the recovery position. Administer oxygen if it is available. Transfer the patient to the hospital emergency department.

Diabetic coma

Diabetic coma is due to an accumulation of glucose and acid by-products in the bloodstream. The patient is hyperglycaemic from having eaten a meal but failed to take the insulin dose. As this form of diabetic coma generally takes several days of dietary and insulin mismanagement before it becomes evident it is unlikely that the patient will present as an emergency during a podiatric surgical treatment. The patient's skin will feel dry and the face flushed, will have deep rapid breathing and the *breath will smell of acetone*

(nail varnish). The patient may complain of thirst, nausea or air hunger and may vomit.

The treatment is to transfer the patient to the hospital emergency department without delay. If the person is unconscious place in the recovery position. Administer oxygen.

TIP: The patient may have a hospital card or be wearing an SOS bracelet.

Asthmatic attack

It is very unlikely that you will have a patient who is unaware that he or she is asthmatic, but the possibility of a stress-related asthmatic attack taking place during a surgical procedure must always be considered.

TIP: Known asthma patients should always take their asthma medication (often in the form of an inhaler) with them into the procedure room.

During an asthmatic attack the patient may have difficulty in breathing (dyspnoea) and the attack may be of gradual or of sudden onset. Often the first complaint is of a feeling of heaviness in the chest. This is often followed by wheezing or coughing. The patient may also become anxious and will sit up or stand 'gasping for air'.

The blood pressure, pulse and respiratory rate will increase. The attack may last from several minutes to, in extreme cases, hours. The patient may use an inhaler, which often ends the attack. In the case of a slight attack prompt use of the inhaler by the patient may be enough to treat the episode.

TIP: With young children, removing the child from the treatment room may be all that is required.

In a severe attack if the patient's own medication is having no noticeable beneficial effect the patient *must be transferred to a hospital*. Whilst waiting for transport the patient should be allowed to get into the most comfortable position, and if there is still no beneficial response from the patient's inhaler then oxygen should be given.

> **TIP:** In a case of status asthmaticus, which is a severe form of asthmatic attack that does not respond to normal medication, consider the possibility of pulmonary or cardiopulmonary arrest.

10

Anatomy of the foot

Podiatric surgical students will have spent some considerable time learning the anatomy of the foot in great detail, whereas podiatric assistants without any previous medical training may have only a limited knowledge of the anatomy of the foot. Therefore it is the intention of this chapter to introduce to the new assistant the terminology, and locations of the various bones and soft tissue structures that podiatrists use in the day-to-day practice of surgery.

BONES OF THE FOOT

Basically each foot consists of 26 bones (Fig. 10.1), and two principal sesamoids, which are found under the first metatarsal head. These 26 bones are divided into three segments as follows.

1. *The posterior segment*; this consists of two bones—the calcaneus and the talus.
2. *The middle segment*; this consists of the five tarsal bones—the navicular, the medial cuneiform, the intermediate cuneiform, the lateral cuneiform and the cuboid.
3. *The anterior segment*; this segment consists of five metatarsals and 14 phalangeal bones. The first or great toe has two phalanges; the other toes have three each.

THE ARTICULATED BONES OF THE FOOT

Figure 10.2 shows the articular bones from the medial and lateral aspects (left).

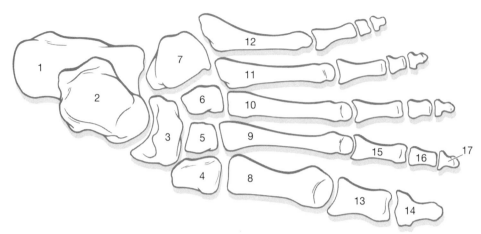

Figure 10.1 Bones of the foot.

Posterior segment
  1. Calcaneus.
  2. Talus.

Middle segment
  3. Navicular.
  4. Medial cuneiform.
  5. Intermediate cuneiform.

  6. Lateral cuneiform.
  7. Cuboid.

Anterior segment
  8. First metatarsal.
  9., 10., 11., 12. Second, third, fourth
    and fifth metatarsals.
  13. Proximal phalanx of the great toe.

  14. Distal phalanx of the great toe.
  15. Proximal phalanx of the second
    toe.
  16. Middle phalanx of the second toe.
  17. Distal phalanx of the second toe.

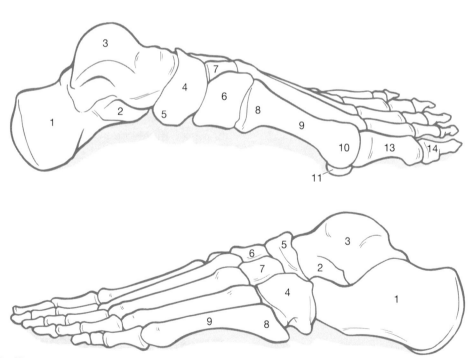

Figure 10.2 The articulated bones of the foot. A: medial and B: lateral aspects.

Figure 10.2 (Cont.)

Medial aspect
1. Calcaneus.
2. Sustentaculum tali.
3. Talus.
4. Navicular.
5. Tuberosity of the navicular.
6. Medial cuneiform.
7. Intermediate cuneiform.
8. Base of first metatarsal.
9. Body of first metatarsal.

10. Head of first metatarsal.
11. Sesamoid bone.
12. Head of second metatarsal.
13. Body of proximal phalanx of great toe.
14. Body of distal phalanx of great toe.

Lateral aspect
1. Calcaneus.
2. Tarsal sinus.
3. Talus.
4. Cuboid.
5. Navicular.
6. Intermediate cuneiform.
7. Lateral cuneiform.
8. Tuberosity of fifth metatarsal.
9. Body of fifth metatarsal.

ANATOMICAL LANDMARKS OF THE FOOT

Dorsum left foot (Fig. 10.3)

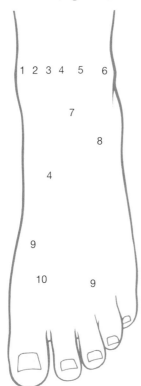

Figure 10.3   Anatomical landmarks of the foot (dorsum left foot).

1. Medial malleolus.
2. Great saphenous vein and nerve.
3. Tibialis anterior.
4. Extensor hallucis longus.
5. Extensor digitorum longus.
6. Lateral malleolus.
7. Anterior tibial artery.
8. Extensor digitorum brevis.
9. Dorsal venous arch.
10. Dorsalis pedis artery.

Rear view left foot (Fig. 10.4)

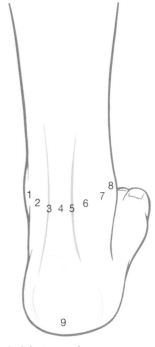

Figure 10.4   Left foot, rear view.

1. Lateral malleolus.
2. Peroneus longus and brevis.
3. Small saphenous vein and sural nerve.
4. Tendo calcaneus.
5. Flexor hallucis longus.
6. Posterior tibial artery and nerve.
7. Flexor digitorum longus and tibial nerve.
8. Medial malleolus.
9. Tuberosity of the calcaneus.

Medial aspect left foot (Fig. 10.5)

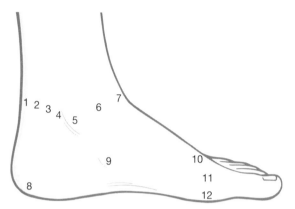

Figure 10.5 Left foot, medial aspect.

1. Tendo calcaneus.
2. Flexor hallucis longus.
3. Posterior tibial artery and nerve.
4. Flexor digitorum longus and tibialis posterior.
5. Medial malleolus.
6. Great saphenous vein and saphenous nerve.
7. Tibialis anterior.
8. Tuberosity of the calcaneus.
9. Tuberosity of the navicular.
10. Extensor hallucis longus.
11. Head of first metatarsal.
12. Sesamoid.

Lateral aspect left foot (Fig. 10.6)

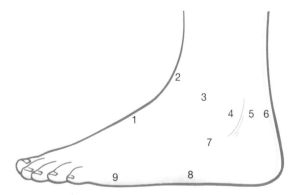

Figure 10.6 Left foot, lateral aspect.

1. Extensor hallucis longus.
2. Tibialis anterior.
3. Extensor digitorum longus.
4. Lateral malleolus.
5. Peroneus longus and brevis.
6. Small saphenous vein and sural nerve.
7. Extensor digitorum brevis.
8. Tuberosity of base of fifth metatarsal.
9. Head of fifth metatarsal.

MUSCLES AND LIGAMENTS AND SYNOVIAL SHEATHS, DORSUM OF FOOT (Fig. 10.7)

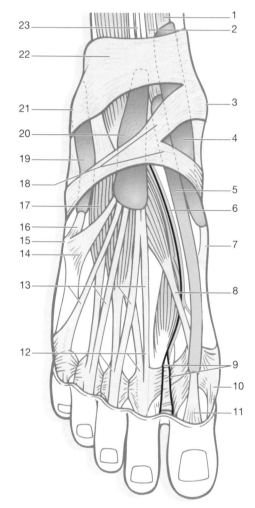

Figure 10.7 Muscles and ligaments and synovial sheaths, dorsum of foot.

1. Tibialis anterior.
2. Extensor hallucis longus.
3. Medial malleolus.
4. Sheath of tibialis anterior.
5. Sheath of extensor hallucis longus.
6. Dorsalis pedis artery.
7. Tibialis anterior.
8. Extensor hallucis brevis.
9. Deep peroneal nerve.
10. Extensor expansion.
11. Extensor hallucis longus.
12. Tendons of extensor digitorum brevis.
13. Tendons of extensor digitorum longus.
14. Peroneus tertius.
15. Tuberosity of fifth metatarsal.

Figure 10.7 (Cont.)
16. Peroneus brevis.
17. Extensor digitorum brevis.
18. Inferior retinaculum.
19. Sheath of peroneal tendons.
20. Sheath of extensor digitorum longus.
21. Lateral malleolus.
22. Superior extensor retinaculum.
23. Extensor digitorum longus.

BONES OF THE FIRST AND SECOND TOES (Fig. 10.8)

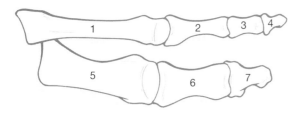

Figure 10.8   Bones of the first and second toes.

1. Second metatarsal.
2. Proximal phalanx.
3. Middle phalanx.
4. Distal phalanx.
5. First metatarsal.
6. Proximal phalanx of the hallux.
7. Distal phalanx.

CAPSULES AND LIGAMENTS OF THE METATARSOPHALANGEAL JOINT AND INTERPHALANGEAL JOINTS (Fig. 10.9)

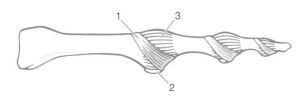

Figure 10.9   Capsules and ligaments of the metatarsophalangeal joint and interphalangeal joints.

1. Collateral ligament.
2. Plantar ligament (plate).
3. Articular capsule.

MUSCLES AND LIGAMENTS OF THE SOLE OF THE FOOT

First layer (Fig. 10.10)

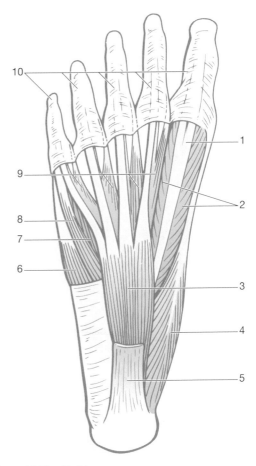

Figure 10.10   First layer.

1. Tendon of flexor hallucis longus.
2. Flexor hallucis brevis.
3. Flexor digitorum brevis.
4. Abductor hallucis.
5. Plantar aponeurosis (cut).
6. Abductor digiti minimi.
7. Plantar interosseous.
8. Flexor digiti minimi brevis.
9. Lumbricales.
10. Digital sheaths.

Second layer (Fig. 10.11)

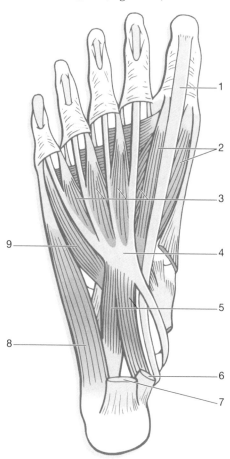

Figure 10.11 Second layer.

1. Tendon of flexor hallucis longus.
2. Flexor hallucis brevis.
3. Lumbricales.
4. Tendon of flexor digitorum longus.
5. Quadratus plantae.
6. Flexor digitorum brevis (cut).
7. Abductor hallucis (cut).
8. Abductor digiti minimi.
9. Flexor digiti minimi brevis.

Third layer (Fig. 10.12)

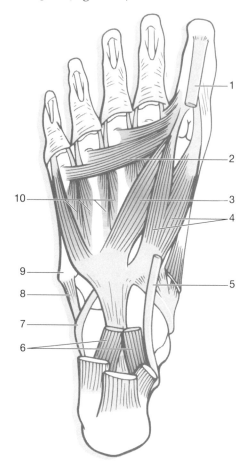

Figure 10.12 Third layer.

1. Flexor hallucis longus (cut).
2. Transverse head of adductor.
3. Oblique head of adductor hallucis.
4. Flexor hallucis brevis.
5. Flexor hallucis longus (cut).
6. Quadratus plantae (cut).
7. Tendon of peroneus longus.
8. Tendon of peroneus brevis.
9. Tuberosity of fifth metatarsal.
10. Plantar interossei.

Fourth layer (Fig. 10.13)

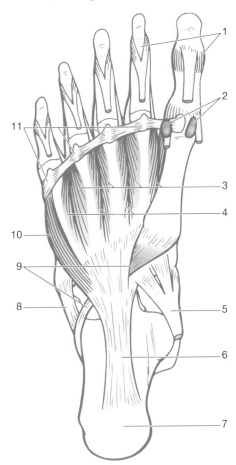

Figure 10.13   Fourth layer.

1. Articular capsule.
2. Sesamoid bones.
3. Dorsal interossei.
4. Plantar interossei.
5. Tendon of tibialis posterior.
6. Long plantar ligament.
7. Calcaneal tuberosity longus.
8. Peroneus brevis tendon.
9. Peroneus longus tendon.
10. Flexor digiti minimi.
11. Plantar ligaments.

BONES OF THE FOOT—PLANTAR VIEW (Fig. 10.14)

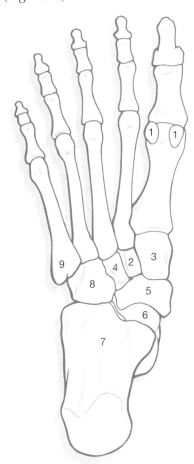

Figure 10.14   Bones of the foot, plantar view.

1. Sesamoid bones.
2. Intermediate cuneiform.
3. Medial cuneiform.
4. Lateral cuneiform.
5. Navicular.
6. Talus.
7. Groove for flexor hallucis.
8. Cuboid.
9. Tuberosity of fifth metatarsal.

MOVEMENTS OF THE FOOT

Dorsiflexion

This is also known as extension (Fig. 10.15).

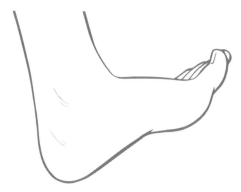

Figure 10.15 Dorsiflexion.

Plantarflexion

This is also known as flexion (Fig. 10.16).

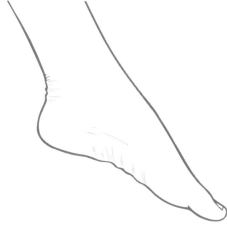

Figure 10.16 Plantarflexion.

Inversion (from the front)

This may also be called adduction (Fig. 10.17).

Eversion (from the front)

This may also be called abduction (Fig. 10.18). (Abduction is also used to describe spreading the toes apart.)

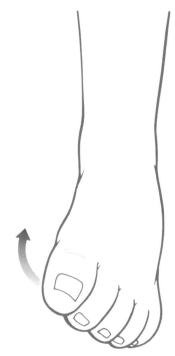

Figure 10.17 Inversion.

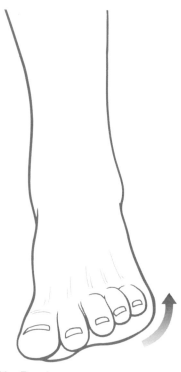

Figure 10.18 Eversion.

11

Forefoot disorders that are suitable for outpatient (office) procedures

The majority of forefoot disorders are suitable for outpatient podiatric surgery, and it is the intention of this section to introduce the assistant and student podiatrist to some of the more common pathologies that will be encountered in day-to-day experience. It is not within the scope of this book to describe the operative details and students are advised to read the appropriate textbooks for details of the operative procedures that are listed for each deformity mentioned in this section.

The operation of choice for each pathology will depend on a number of factors such as:

• severity of the deformity
• cause of the deformity
• medical condition, and history of the patient
• expectations of the patient
• associated secondary complications that may occur after a specific procedure; as an example, after the amputation of the second toe, a hallux valgus deformity may result
• choice of the surgeon, based on the above, but also to some extent on the surgeon's own training and previous experience of the different procedures; for example, there are very many procedures for the treatment of hallux valgus, and the one chosen may well be based to a large extent on the surgeon's clinical experience in relation to a particular procedure.

HAMMER TOE

This is shown in Figure 11.1.

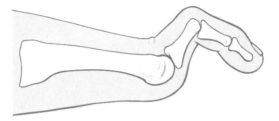

Figure 11.1 Hammer toe.

Procedures that may be employed for hammer toe include:

- amputation
- arthrodesis (spike or peg)
- arthroplasty—head of proximal phalanx
- arthroplasty—base of proximal phalanx
- capsulotomy—metatarsophalangeal joint
- tenotomy—extensor tendons.

Note that amputation of the second toe may result in a hallux valgus deformity. Arthroplasty of the base of the proximal phalanx often gives a good result in the first instance but in the long term it may result in destabilization of the toe with dorsal displacement of the toe as the adjacent toes come together.

MALLET TOE

This is shown in Figure 11.2.

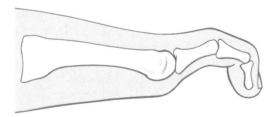

Figure 11.2 Mallet toe.

Procedures that may be employed for mallet toe include:

- amputation of distal phalanx
- arthrodesis—middle and distal phalanx

- arthroplasty—head of middle phalanx (in this procedure it is recommended that the flexor tendon is also cut, between the head of the middle phalanx and base of the distal phalanx)
- total excision of the middle phalanx.

SWAN NECK TOE

This is shown in Figure 11.3.

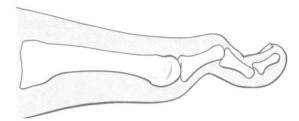

Figure 11.3 Swan neck toe.

Procedures that may be employed for swan neck toe include:

- arthrodesis
- arthroplasty
- tenotomy
- total excision of middle phalanx.

The severity of the deformity may necessitate a combination of all or some of the above procedures.

CLAW TOE (RETRACTED)

This may be due to a subluxed proximal phalanx. It is shown in Figure 11.4.

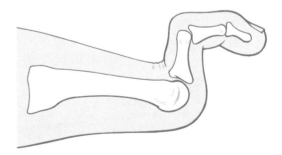

Figure 11.4 Claw toe (retracted): subluxed proximal phalanx.

Procedures that may be employed for claw toe include:

- amputation
- arthroplasty—base of proximal phalanx
- capsulotomy—metatarsophalangeal joint
- tenotomy—extensor tendons
- combination of arthroplasty, tenotomy and capsulotomy.

HYPEREXTENSION OF THE HALLUX

This is shown in Figure 11.5.

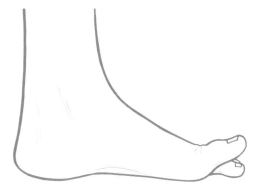

Figure 11.5 Hyperextension of the hallux.

Procedures that may be employed for hyperextension of the hallux include:

- arthrodesis of metatarsal and proximal phalanx
- capsulotomy—metatarsophalangeal joint
- Keller's arthroplasty (if not the cause)
- VY plasty, often in combination with a Z plasty
- Z plasty—extensor tendon.

HALLUX RIGIDUS (DORSAL BUNION)

This is shown in Figure 11.6.

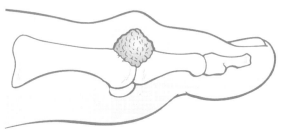

Figure 11.6 Hallux rigidus (dorsal bunion).

Procedures that may be employed for hallux rigidus include:

- cheilectomy (reduction of osteophytic lipping)
- Keller's arthroplasty (patients over 60)
- Silver's bunionectomy for medial exostosis
- simple reduction of dorsal exostosis
- Valanti procedure.

HALLUX FLEXUS (TRIGGER TOE)

This may be due to a subluxated proximal phalanx. It is shown in Figure 11.7.

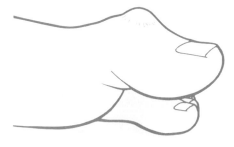

Figure 11.7 Hallux flexus (trigger toe).

Procedures that may be employed for hallux flexus include:

- arthrodesis
- arthroplasty—proximal phalanx
- capsulotomy—metatarsophalangeal joint
- Keller's arthroplasty
- VY plasty
- Z plasty of extensor tendon
- combination of the above.

OVERRIDING SECOND TOE AND HALLUX VALGUS

This is shown in Figure 11.8.

Procedures that may be employed for overriding second toe include:

- amputation of second toe
- arthrodesis of second toe in combination with a bunion procedure
- arthroplasty of second toe in combination with a Keller's arthroplasty
- Keller's arthroplasty.

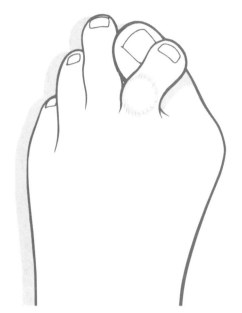

Figure 11.8 Overriding second toe and hallux valgus.

OVERLAPPING FIFTH TOE (ADDUCTOVARUS DEFORMITY)

This is shown in Figure 11.9.

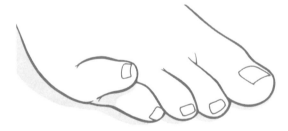

Figure 11.9 Overlapping fifth toe (adductovarus deformity).

Procedures that may be employed for overriding fifth toe include:

- amputation
- arthrodesis
- arthroplasty
- capsulotomy—metatarsophalangeal joint
- chevron—proximal phalanx (Austin)
- syndactyly
- syndactyly in combination with arthroplasty of base of proximal phalanx
- tenotomy
- VY plasty
- VY plasty in combination with tenotomy
- combination of the above.

TAILOR'S BUNION (BUNIONETTE)

This is shown in Figure 11.10.

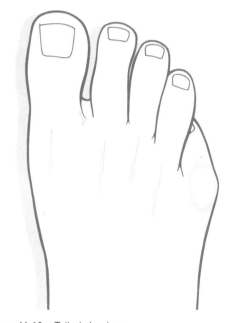

Figure 11.10 Tailor's bunion.

Procedures that may be employed for Tailor's bunion include:

- amputation of fifth toe (not recommended)
- arthroplasty base of proximal phalanx of fifth toe (if there is no varus deformity at the head of the proximal phalanx)
- arthrodesis (not recommended as the rigid toe can rub on the shoe)
- capsulotomy—metatarsophalangeal joint
- chevron procedure—head of fifth metatarsal
- oblique osteotomy—fifth metatarsal shaft
- simple reduction of exostosis (lateral aspect of metatarsal head).

HALLUX VALGUS (MILD)

This is shown in Figure 11.11.

Procedures that may be employed for mild hallux valgus include:

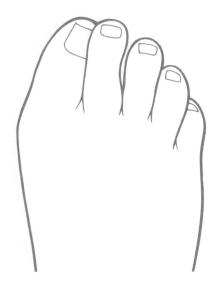

Figure 11.11 Hallux valgus (mild).

- Akin—closing wedge osteotomy, base of proximal phalanx of the hallux
- chevron osteotomy (Austin)
- McBride or modified McBride
- Silver's bunionectomy (if a medial exostosis is present)
- Wilson osteotomy.

HALLUX VALGUS (MODERATE)

This is shown in Figure 11.12.

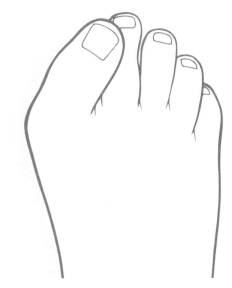

Figure 11.12 Hallux valgus (moderate).

Procedures that may be employed for moderate hallux valgus include:

- Keller's arthroplasty
- Wilson osteotomy
- various osteotomies, although most are not suitable for outpatient procedures.

Abbreviations and symbols used in podiatric surgery

Ideally abbreviations should not be used, but are! Some are international and some are confined to specific podiatry schools and hospitals. Below are a list of the more common ones found in general podiatry.

A

A/	apex, e.g. A/3 = apex of third toe
A & E	Accident and Emergency Department (ER in USA)
AF	atrial fibrillation
AFO	ankle foot orthotic
AIDS	acquired immune deficiency syndrome
ANT	anterior
AP	anteroposterior (radiograph)
APMA	American Podiatric Medical Association
AROM	active range of motion
AT	anterior tibial pulse

B

B/F	both feet
BLS	basic life support
BNF	British National Formulary
BP	blood pressure/British Pharmacopoeia
BPC	British Pharmacopoeia
BS	blood sugar

C

C	Centigrade
c̄	with
Cal	callus
CBC	complete blood count
C/C	chief complaint

CHD	congenital heart disease
Chr	chiropody
cm	centimetre
CNS	central nervous system
C/O	complains of
CO_2	carbon dioxide
CPMA	callus plantar metatarsal area
CPR	cardiopulmonary resuscitation
Cres	crescent pad
C & S	culture and sensitivity
cu mm	cubic millimetre
CVA	cerebrovascular accident

D

DIPJ	distal interphalangeal joint
DIST	distal
DJD	degenerative joint disease
DNA	patient did not attend
DNKA	did not keep appointment
DOB	date of birth
Dor	dorsal
DP	dorsiplantar view (radiograph)
DP	dorsalis pedis (pulse)
DPM	Doctor of Podiatric Medicine (US)
D.Pod.M.	Diploma in Podiatric Medicine (UK)
DVT	deep vein thrombosis

E

ECG	electrocardiogram
EEG	electroencephalogram
ER	emergency room (US) (= A & E in UK)
ESR	erythrocyte sedimentation rate

F

F	Fahrenheit
F/	feet
Ft	foot
FTA	failed to attend
FB	foreign body
FBC	full blood count
FBS	fasting blood sugar
FCA	footcare assistant
Fib	fibula

G

GA	general anaesthetic
GHG	general health good
GI	gastrointestinal
g	gram
GP	general practitioner
GT	green towel
GTT	glucose tolerance test

H

Θ	haemorrhage
HAV	hallux abducto valgus
Hb	haemoglobin
HBP	high blood pressure
HD	heloma durum
HEM	haemorrhage
HG	hypergranulation tissue
Hg	mercury
HIB	Hibitane® (chlorhexidine)
HIV	human immunodeficiency virus
HL	hallux limitus
HM	heloma molle
Hmill	seed corn
HNV	neurovascular corn
H/O	history of
HPC	history of presenting complaint
HR	hallux rigidus
HRT	hormone replacement therapy
HT	hammer toe
H/T	hypertension
HV	hallux valgus
H Vasc	vascular corn

I

ID	infectious disease
ID/	interdigital, e.g. ID 1/2
IDDM	insulin-dependent diabetes mellitus
IDW	interdigital wedge
IM	intermetatarsal
IMA	intermetatarsal angle
IMS	industrial methylated spirit
in	inch
INF	inferior
INJT	injection
IPJ	interphalangeal joint
IU	international unit
IV	intravenous

J

Jt (J)	joint

K

K	potassium
Kg	kilogram

L

LA	local anaesthesia
LAT	lateral
LBP	low back pain
LE	lupus erythematosus
LF	left foot

LIG	ligament
LMN	lower motor neuron
LO	lateral oblique (radiograph)
LOM	limitation of motion
L–R	left to right
LV	left ventricle
LVF	left ventricle failure

M

M	male
MAN	manipulation
MAOI	monoamine oxidase inhibitors
MCH	mean corpuscular haemoglobin
MCHC	mean corpuscular haemoglobin concentration
MChS	Member of the Society of Chiropodists and Podiatrists (UK)
MCV	mean corpuscular volume
MED	medial
MET	metatarsal
mg	milligram
MI	myocardial infarction
MID	middle
ml	millilitre
mm	millimetre
MRI	magnetic resonance imaging
MS	multiple sclerosis
MSU	midstream (urine)
MT	metatarsal
MTJ	midtarsal joint
MTPJ	metatarsophalangeal joint

N

N/A	non-applicable
Na	sodium
NAD	no abnormalities detected
NBI	no bone injury
neg.	negative
NFV	no further visit
NHS	National Health Service
NIDDM	non-insulin-dependent diabetes mellitus
N/K	not known
NM	neuromuscular
NSAID	non-steroidal anti-inflammatory drug
NWB	non-weight-bearing
NYD	not yet diagnosed

O

O_2	oxygen
OA	osteoarthritis
OC	onychocryptosis (ingrowing toe nail)
OCP	oval cavity pad

O/E	on examination
OG	onychogryphosis
O/H	subungual corn
OMYC	onychomycosis
OP	operation/onychophosis
OR	operating room (US) (= operating theatre UK)
OX	onychauxis

P

PA	Podiatry Association
PC	presenting complaint
PCV	packed cell volume
PE	pulmonary embolus
PIPJ	proximal interphalangeal joint
PL	plantar
PMH	previous medical history
PMP	plantar metatarsal pad
PNA	partial nail avulsion
POP	plaster of Paris
PP	pre- and postoperative/pressure point
PROX	proximal
PT	posterior tibial pulse
PVD	peripheral vascular disease

R

R/	right foot
RA	rheumatoid arthritis
RBC	red blood cell
RBS	random blood sugar
RDW	red cell distribution width
RF	right foot
R–L	right to left
ROM	range of motion
RTA	road traffic accident

S

SBE	subacute bacterial endocarditis
SCF	semicompressed felt
SRCh	State Registered Chiropodist (UK)
STJ	subtalar joint
SUB	beneath
SUBQ	subcutaneous tissue
Sub Ung	subungual
SUP	superior
SWG	standard wire gauge

T

TAB	tablet
TB	Tailor's bunion/tuberculosis
T & C	tenotomy and capsulotomy
TCJ	talocrural joint

TEMP	temperature		VU	varicose ulcer
TENS	transcutaneous electrical nerve stimulation		VV	varicose vein(s)
TF	tube foam			
TG	tube gauze		**W**	
TIA	transient ischaemic attack		WB	weight-bearing
TNA	total nail avulsion		WBC	white blood cell (count)
TP	tibial posterior pulse		WNL	within normal limits
			WT	weight
U				
UA	urinalysis		**Y**	
U & E	urea and electrolytes		YOB	year of birth
UMN	upper motor neuron			
UNG	ointment		<<	condition deteriorated
US	ultrasound		>>	condition improved
U/S	unserviceable		#	number/fracture
USP	United States Pharmacopeia		<	less than
			>	more than
V			≤	equal to or less than
VAS	visual analogue scale		≥	equal to or more than
VD	venereal disease		±	plus or minus
VF	ventricular fibrillation		§	section
VS	vital signs		≅	approximately equal to
			Δ	diagnosis

Appendix 2

Glossary

Like any other profession podiatry has its own vocabulary, and podiatrists may use words that are unfamiliar to you as a new assistant who has no previous medical knowledge. Therefore, to assist you in the front-office duties of the recording of the patient's charts and letter writing, the following is a glossary of some of the more common words used in podiatric surgery, together with their phonetic pronunciation and alternative spellings.

Abduct (ab-dukt') To draw away from the median plane or (in the toes) from the axial line of the limb.

Abscess (ab'-ses) A cavity with an accumulation of pus.

Achilles tendon (a-kil'ez) Tendo calcaneus, the tendon of the muscles of the calf of the leg (the gastrocnemius and soleus muscles).

Acromegaly (ak'-ro-meg'ah-le) Abnormal growth of the hands, feet and face, caused by hypersecretion of the pituitary gland.

Adduct (ad-dukt') To draw towards the median plane or (in the toes) towards the axial line of the limb.

Adhesion (ad-he'zhun) The union of surfaces due to inflammation. *Primary adhesion*—healing by first intention. *Secondary adhesion*—healing by second intention.

Adrenaline The British Pharmacopoeia name for epinephrine.

Allergy A hypersensitive state acquired through exposure to a particular allergen.

Ampoule/ampule (am'pul)   A small sealed capsule holding specified quantities of drugs, especially for injecting.

Anaemia/anemia   Deficiency in the blood, usually of red cells or their haemoglobin.

Anaesthesia/anesthesia (an'es-the'ze-ah)   Loss of feeling or sensation, especially the loss of pain sensation induced to allow surgery.

Anaesthetic/anesthetic (an'-nes'thet'ik)   An agent that produces anaesthesia.

Analgesia   The absence of normal sensation of pain.

Analgesic   A drug that relieves pain.

Anaphylaxis (an-a-fil-ak'-sis)   A severe reaction, occasionally fatal, resulting from injection of a substance to which an individual has become sensitized; also called *anaphylactic shock*.

Aneurysm/aneurism (an'-u-rizm)   Localized enlargement of an artery.

Angina pectoris (an-ji'nah)   Severe pain and constriction around the heart, usually radiating to the left shoulder and down the left arm.

Ankylosis/anchylosis   Immobility of a joint due to disease or a planned surgical procedure.

Anterior (an-te're-or)   Situated or directed towards the front.

Antibiotic (an'ti-bi-ot'ik)   An agent derived from a microorganism, which has the capacity to inhibit the growth or to kill other microorganisms.

Anticoagulant (an'ti-ko-ag'u-lant)   A drug that prevents clotting of blood.

Antisepsis (an'ti-sep'sis)   Prevention of sepsis.

Antiseptic (an'ti-sep'tik)   Any agent that prevents the growth of organisms causing sepsis in wounds.

Apex   The top or pointed end of a structure.

Arterial (ar-te're-al)   Relating to an artery.

Arteriole   A minute artery that leads into a capillary.

Arteriolosclerosis (ar-te're-o'lo-skle-ro'sis)   Thickening of the walls of arteries with loss of elasticity.

Artery   A vessel carrying blood from the heart.

Arthrectomy   Excision of a joint.

Arthritis   Inflammation of a joint.

Arthrodesis   Surgical fusion of a joint.

Arthroplasty (ar'thro-plas'te)   An operation to reshape or reconstruct a diseased or damaged joint.

Arthrotome   An instrument for making incisions into a joint.

Arthrotomy (ar-throt'o-me)   An incision into a joint.

Asepsis (a-sep'sis)   Sterile; a condition free from pathogenic microorganisms.

Aspirate (as'pi-rat)   To draw out by suction.

Astringent   An agent that checks haemorrhage.

Athlete's foot   A fungus infection of the foot between the toes caused by various dermatophytes, especially *Trichophyton rubrum, Trichophyton metagrophytes* and *Epidermophyton fioccosun*; medical name *tinea pedis*.

Atrophy (at'ro-fe)   A wasting or shrinking in size of any organ or tissue.

Autoclave (aw'to'klav)   A sterilizer using high-pressure steam.

Avulsion   The forceful tearing away of tissue.

Babinski's reflex   Present in disease or injury to the upper motor neuron. *See* Plantar reflex.

Bacteria   Any disease-producing microorganism of the class Schizomycetes.

Bactericide (bak-ter'-i-sid)   An agent that destroys bacteria.

Basophil (ba'so-fil)   Cells that are readily stained with basic dyes such as methylene blue.

Beau's lines   Transverse lines across the nails. May be an indication of systemic disease.

Benign   Non-malignant.

Bilateral (bi-lat'er-al)   Affecting two sides.

Biomechanics (bi-'o-me-kan'iks)   The study of the mechanical laws relating to the movement or structure of living organisms.

Biopsy (bi'op-se)   Examination of tissue to discover the presence or cause of disease.

Bleb   A small swelling under or on the skin.

Blood count   The number of the red corpuscles and the leucocytes per mm^3 of whole blood.

Boil   An inflamed area of the skin containing pus. Medical name *furuncle*.

Bradycardia   Slowing of the heart rate to less than 60 beats per minute.

Brodie's abscess   An abscess of the head of the tibia. A form of chronic tuberculous or staphylococcal osteomyelitis.

Bruise A contusion, a superficial injury to the tissue caused by a sudden impact in which the skin is unbroken.

Bulla A blister containing serous fluid, larger than a vesicle.

Bunion (bun'-yun) A prominence of the first metatarsal joint; it may also include a bursa and abnormal alignment of the first metatarsophalangeal joint.

Bunionectomy (bun'yun-ek'to-me) The excision of a bunion.

Bunionette (bun'yun-et') Enlargement of the lateral aspect of the fifth metatarsal head; also called *Tailor's bunion.*

Bursa (ber'-sah) A small sac of fibrous tissue lined with a synovial membrane and filled with fluid; also called *synovia.*

Bursitis (ber'si'tis) Inflammation of a bursa.

Calcaneal spur An outgrowth on the base or back of the calcaneum.

Calcaneus/os calcis (kal-ka'ne-us) Heel bone, calcaneum.

Callosity A hard area of skin occurring on parts of the foot subject to friction or pressure.

Callus (kal'us) A mass of granulation tissue and blood containing bone-forming cells that forms around the ends of bones after a fracture.

Cannula A flexible sheath enclosing a trocar, the tube allowing the escape of fluid after the trocar is withdrawn.

Cannulation Introduction of a cannula.

Capsule (kap'su-l) The two-layered covering of a synovial joint. The inner layer is synovial and the outer is fibrous.

Capsulitis (kap'su-li'tis) Inflammation of a capsule.

Capsulotomy ((kap'su-lot'o-me) The cutting into a capsule.

Cartilage (articular) (kar'ti-lij) The covering for the articular surface of bones; also called *hyaline cartilage.*

Cauterize/cauterise (kaw'ter-ise) Coagulate tissue with heat.

Cheilectomy Surgical removal of a lip of bone around a joint in order to facilitate joint mobility.

Chilblain A condition resulting from defective circulation, characterized by localized erythema.

The area itches, and may become painful; medical name *pernio.*

Chlorhexidine An antiseptic used as a general disinfectant for skin; trade name *Hibitane*®.

Chondritis Inflammation of cartilage.

Chondroma A benign growth arising in cartilage.

Claudication Lameness. *Intermittent claudication*— limping, accompanied by severe pain in the legs on walking; disappears with rest.

Coalesce To fuse a joint. Noun *coalition.*

Collateral ligaments Ligaments connecting bones to each other.

Condyle (kon'-dil) A rounded eminence occurring at the end of some bones.

Condylectomy Excision of a condyle.

Congenital (kon-jen'i-tal) Present at birth.

Contusion (kon-too'zhun) A bruise.

Convulsion Spasmodic contractions of muscles.

Crepitation (krep-it-a'-shun) The grating sound caused by friction of the two ends of a fractured bone.

Cryosurgery Surgery using the local application of intense cold.

Cuboid bone Outer bone of the tarsal bones articulating posteriorly with the fourth and fifth metatarsals.

Curette (ku-ret) A spoon-shaped instrument used for scraping bone.

Cutaneous (ku-ta'ne-us) Pertaining to the skin.

Cyanosis The bluish discoloration of the skin caused by poor oxygenation of the blood.

Cyst A closed sac, with a definite wall that contains fluid or semifluid material.

Debridement The cleaning of an open wound by removal of foreign or dead tissue to promote healing.

Defibrillation (de-fib-ril-a-shun) The restoration of normal rhythm to the heart in ventricular fibrillation by means of high voltage.

Defibrillator (de-fib-ril-a'-tor) An electrical device by which normal rhythm is restored in ventricular fibrillation.

Dermatitis Inflammation of the skin.

Dermatocyst A skin cyst.

Dermatome The area of skin supplied with afferent nerve fibres by a single posterior spinal root.

Diagnosis Determination of the nature of a disease.

Diathermy (di-a-ther'-me) Production of heat by high-frequency electric current. *Surgical diathermy*—current of very high frequency, used to coagulate blood vessels or dissect tissue.

Dislocation (dis-lo-ka'-shun) The displacement of a bone from its natural position.

Distal Further from a point of reference.

Dorsal Relating to the back of an object or organ.

Dorsalis pedis pulse A pulse on the dorsal aspect of the foot.

Dorsiflexion To bend the foot backwards (the toes upwards).

Dorsum The upper or posterior surface.

Dyspnoea/dyspnea (disp-ne-ah) Breathlessness.

Ecchymosis (ek-ke-mo'sis) A discoloration of the skin caused by the extravasation of blood.

Eczema (ek'-ze-mah) An acute or chronic inflammatory condition of the skin.

Embolism (em'bo'lizm) The sudden blocking of an artery by a clot or foreign material.

Eosinophil A cell that has an affinity for acid stains.

Epidermis The outer layer of skin.

Epidermoid cyst A cyst within the epidermis.

Epinephrine (ep-e-nef'-rin) US Pharmacopeia name for adrenaline.

Eponychium (ep'-o-nik'e-um) The fold of epidermis that overlaps the base of the nail.

Equinus The foot in a plantar-flexed position.

Erythema A superficial redness of the skin.

Erythema ab igne Localized erythema caused by exposure to heat, occasionally seen on the legs of elderly people who sit in front of open fires.

Erythrocyte Red blood cells.

Esmarch's bandage (es'mark) A rubber bandage that is applied tightly to the limb, commencing at the distal end and reaching above the site of operation where a tourniquet is then applied. The Esmarch's bandage is then removed, rendering the surgical site a virtually bloodless area.

Eversion Turning outwards.

Excise (eks-siz') To remove (by cutting).

Excision To surgically remove a structure or organ by cutting.

Exostosis (eks-os-to'-sis) A benign cartilaginous outgrowth from a bone.

Exsanguinate (eks-san-gwin-at') To deprive an area of blood; *see also* Esmarch's bandage.

Extension The act of extending a joint.

Extensor (eks-ten'sor) A muscle that extends a part; *see also* Hallucis brevis, Hallucis longus.

Extravasation The escape of fluids into the surrounding tissue.

Fascia (fash'e-ah) A sheath of connective tissue, enclosing muscle.

Femoral Pertaining to the femur or to the thigh.

Fibre/fiber An elongated threadlike structure.

Fibroma (fi-bro'-mah) A benign tumour of fibrous tissue.

Fibula (fib'-u-lah) The slender bone on the outer side of the leg.

First intention Healing that takes place without granulation tissue having been formed.

Fissure (fish'-ur) A groove or cleft-like defect in the skin.

Flexor (flek'ser) Any muscle that flexes a joint.

Foramen (fo-ra'men) A natural opening into bone. *Nutrient foramen*—any of the passages admitting nutrient vessels to the medullary cavity of bone.

Forceps (for'seps) An instrument designed to grasp an object so it can be held or pulled.

Forefoot valgus Eversion of the distal one-half of the foot.

Forefoot varus Inversion of the distal one-half of the foot.

Formol–saline A formaldehyde solution with saline. Used in histology for tissue preservation.

Fracture A breaking of a part, especially a bone.

Freiberg's infarction Osteochondritis of the head of the second metatarsal.

Fulguration (ful-gur-a'shun) Destruction of tissue by means of high-frequency electric sparks.

Furuncle (fur-unk'-l) 'Boil', a painful nodule formed in the skin.

Fusion (fu'zhun) The operative formation of an ankylosis.

Ganglion (gang'gle-on)   An abnormal harmless swelling that forms within tendon sheaths.

Gangrene (gang'green)   Death of tissue.

Gauze   A thin open-weave material used in the preparation of surgical swabs.

Gentamicin   An antibiotic used to treat infections caused by a wide range of bacteria.

Genu valgum   *'Knock knee'*, a condition in which the knees are close together and the ankles are apart.

Genu varum   *'Bowleg'*, a congenital curvature of the leg, resulting in the knees being abnormally apart, and the ankles abnormally together.

Germicide (jerm'-e-side)   An agent capable of destroying microbes and their spores.

Glucose   An absorbable sugar to which carbohydrates are reduced by digestion, and is therefore found in the blood. It is present in the urine of untreated diabetes mellitus patients.

Granulation tissue (gran-u-la'-shun)   The growth of new tissue in a wound that is not healing by first intention.

Haematoma/hematoma (he-mat-o'-mah)   *'Blood blister'*, an accumulation of blood within the tissues that usually clots.

Haemolysis/hemolysis (he-mol'-is-is)   The destruction of red blood cells.

Haemosiderosis/hemosiderosis (he-mo-sid-er-o'-sis)   The deposition of iron in the tissues as brownish granules following excessive haemolysis of red blood cells.

Haemostasis/hemostasis (he-mo-sta'-sis)   The arrest of bleeding, for example by the application of ligatures.

Haemostat/hemostat   Forceps designed to clamp blood vessels.

Hallucis brevis   The shorter extensor tendon that dorsiflexes the hallux.

Hallucis longus   The tendon and long extensor muscle of the hallux.

Hallux   The great/first/big toe.

Hallux adductus   The displacement of the great toe towards the midline of the body.

Hallux rigidus   Limitation of movement at the metatarsophalangeal joint of the great toe in flexion.

Hallux valgus   The displacement of the great toe away from the midline at the metatarsophalangeal joint.

Hammer toe   A flexion deformity of the proximal interphalangeal joint.

Heloma durum   A hard corn.

Heloma molle   A soft corn that may occur between the digits.

Hemiphalangectomy   Excision of part of a phalanx.

Hexachlorophane   An antiseptic agent, available as a dusting powder; trade names *Dermalex®*, *pHisotlex®*.

Hypertension (hi-per-ten'-shun)   *'High blood pressure'*, an elevation of the arterial blood pressure above the normal range.

Hypertrophy (hi-per'-tro-fe)   Excessive thickening of a part of an organ by increase of its own tissue.

Hypoproteinaemia (hi-po-pro-tin-e'-me-ah)   A deficiency of serum proteins in the blood.

Hypotension (hi-po-ten'-shun)   A low blood pressure.

Ibuprofen   An analgesic that relieves inflammation.

Incision (in-siz'shun)   The surgical cutting of skin.

Infection (in-fek'-shun)   Invasion of the body by harmful organisms (pathogens) such as bacteria or viruses.

Inflammation (in-flam-mai'-shun)   The defensive reaction of tissue to any injury, involving redness, heat, pain, swelling and loss of function of the affected part.

Injection (in-jek'-shun)   The introduction of fluids into the body by means of a syringe.

Intermetatarsal   Between the metatarsal bones.

Intermittent claudication   *See* Claudication.

Interphalangeal   Between the phalanges.

Inversion   Turn towards the midline of the body.

Involuted nail   The edges of the nail turned towards the midline of the toe.

Ischaemia/ischemia (is-ke'-me-ah)   An inadequate flow of blood to a part of the body or an organ.

Keller's operation   An operation to correct a bunion.

Keloid (ke'-loid)   A prominent irregular scar tissue in the skin.

Keratin (ker'-a-tin) A fibrous protein that forms horny tissue, such as toe nails and hair.

Keratoma (ker-a-to'-mah) An overgrowth of horny tissue.

Kirschner wire/K wire (kirsh'-ner) A wire or pin used for the fixation of bone.

Köhler's disease Inflammation of the navicular bone; in children of 3–5 years also called *osteochondritis*.

Laceration (las-er-a'-shun) A wound with torn, ragged edges.

Lateral Pertaining to the side, away from the midline.

Lesion (le'zhun) Any pathological or traumatic alteration in the structure or function of a tissue or organ.

Leucocyte/leukocyte (lu'-ko-site) White blood cell.

Leuconychia/leukonychia (lu-kon-ik'-e-ah) White patches on nails.

Leucopenia/leukopenia (lu-ko-pe'-ne-ah) A decreased number of white cells, usually granulocytes.

Leukaemia/leukemia (lu-ke'-me-ah) A malignant proliferation of blood leucocytes.

Ligament (lig'a-ment) A band of fibrous tissue connecting bones or cartilage, serving to support and strengthen joints.

Ligate (li'gat) To apply a ligature.

Ligation (li-ga'shun) Application of a ligature.

Ligature (lig'ah-tur) Any material used for tying a vessel or to constrict a part.

Lignocaine/lidocaine A local anaesthetic; trade name *Xylocaine*®.

Lipoma (li-po'mah) A benign fatty tumour usually composed of mature fat cells.

Lipping (lip'ing) The development of a bony overgrowth beyond the joint margin in osteoarthritis.

Lunula (lu'nu-lah) The white crescent-shaped area at the base of a nail.

Maceration (mas-er-a'shun) The softening of tissue, noticeably between the toes.

Macrocyte (mak'-ro-site) Abnormally large red corpuscle found in the blood in some forms of anaemia.

Macula/macule (mak'-u-lah) Flat, circumscribed, discoloured lesions of varying shapes and size, not raised above the skin.

Malignant tumour (mal-ig'-nant) A tumour that invades and destroys the tissue and which can spread to other sites in the body, tending to become progressively worse and to result in death.

Malleolus (mal-le-o'-lus) One of the two protuberances on each side of the ankle.

Mallet toe A flexion contracture of the distal interphalangeal joint in the lesser toes.

March fracture A fracture of a metatarsal that occurs without direct pressure; also called *stress fracture*.

Medial (me'de-al) Pertaining to or situated in the midline of a body.

Melanin (mel'ah-nin) A dark pigment.

Melanoma (mel'ah-no'mah) Any tumour composed of melanin-pigmented cells, especially a highly malignant tumour of melanin-forming cells.

Metastasis The spread of a malignant tumour from its site of origin to any other part of the body.

Metatarsal (met'ah-tar'sal) One of the five bones of the metatarsus.

Metatarsal arch The metatarsal bones that make up the transverse arch.

Metatarsalgia Pain in the anterior portion of the metatarsus.

Metatarsophalangeal (met'a-tar'so-fa-lan'je-al) Concerning the metatarsus and phalanges of the toes.

Metatarsus (met'a-tar'-sus) The five bones of the foot uniting the tarsus with the phalanges of the toes.

Microbiology (mi'kro-bi-ol'o-je) The science dealing in the study of microorganisms.

Mole An area of pigment growth; some moles can become malignant; medical name *nevocytic naevus*.

Monocyte A white blood cell having one nucleus, derived from the reticulocyte cells, having a phagocytic action.

Morton's neuroma A neuroma-like mass of the neurovascular bundle of the intermetatarsal spaces, often between the second and third metatarsal heads.

Mycosis (mi-ko'sis) Any disease caused by a fungus.

Myectomy (mi-ek'to-me) A surgical procedure to remove part of a muscle.

Myeloma (mi-e-lo'ma)   A malignant tumour originating in bone marrow.

Narcotic (nar-kot'ic)   A drug that induces stupor and/or insensibility.

Navicular (nah-vik'u-ler)   Boat-shaped bone that articulates with the three cuneiform bones in front and the talus behind.

Necrosis (ne-kro'sis)   Localized death of areas of tissue or bone surrounded by healthy tissue; also called *gangrene*.

Neoplasm (ne'o-plazm)   An abnormal formation of tissue that may be benign or malignant.

Nerve block   A method of producing regional anaesthesia in a part of the body by use of a local anaesthetic.

Neuralgia   Severe pain along the course of a nerve.

Neuritis (nu-ri'tis)   Inflammation of a nerve.

Neuropathy   Any disease of the peripheral nerves, causing weakness or numbness.

Neutrophil (nu'tro-fil)   A leucocyte that stains easily with neutral dyes.

Naevus/nevus (ne'vus)   A congenital discoloration of skin due to pigmentation; *see also* Mole.

Nodule (nod'-ule)   A small swelling or protuberance similar to a papule but larger.

Oblique (o-bleek')   Slanting, diagonal.

Oedema/edema (e-de'-mah)   Excessive accumulation of fluid in the tissues.

Onychectomy (on'i-kek'to-me)   The excision of a nail.

Onychia (o-nik'e-ah)   Inflammation of the nail bed with suppuration; also called *onyxitis*.

Onychocryptosis   Ingrowing toe nail; also called *onyxis*.

Onychodystrophy (on'-i-ko-dis'tro-fe)   A malformation of a nail.

Onychograph (on-ik'o-graf)   An instrument for measuring capillary circulation under the finger nails.

Onychogryphosis (on'i-ko-gri-po'sis)   *'Ram's horn nail'*, abnormal thickening and curvature of the nail.

Onycholysis (oni'-kol'i-sis)   Separation or loosening of part or all of the nail, from the distal edge.

Onychoma (on-i-ko'ma)   A tumour of the nail bed.

Onychomadesis (on'i-ko-ma-de'sis)   Loss of the nail, from the proximal edge.

Onychomalacia   Softening of the nail; also called *hapalonychia*.

Onychomycosis (on'i-ko-mi-ko'sis)   Any fungal disease of a nail.

Onychopathy (on-i-kop'ath-e)   Any disease of the nails; also called *onychosis*.

Onychophosis (on'ik-o-fo'sis)   An accumulation of horny layers of epidermis under the nail.

Onychoptosis   The shedding of the nails.

Onychorrhexis (on'i-ko-rek'sis)   Abnormal brittleness and splitting of the nail plate with longitudinal striations.

Onychoschizia   Loosening and separation of the nail from its bed; also called *onycholysis*.

Orthosis   A device used to correct malalignment of joints, especially those on the foot, to provide support for ambulation, reduce pain and assist motion; adjective *orthotic*.

Orthotics (or-thot'iks)   The science pertaining to mechanical devices or appliances used for the correction of joints.

Orthotist (or'tho-tist)   A specialist in the use and manufacture of orthotic devices.

Ossification   The conversion of tissue into bone.

Ossify (os'ifi)   To develop into bone.

Ostalgia/ostealgia   Pain in the bone.

Ostectomy/osteectomy (os-tek'to-me)   The excision of a bone or part of a bone.

Osteitis (os-te-i'tis)   Inflammation of a bone.

Ostemia (os'te'me-a)   An abnormal congestion of blood in a bone.

Ostempyesis (os'tem-pi-e'sis)   Suppuration within a bone.

Osteoarthritis (os'te-o-ar-thri'tis)   A chronic disease involving the joints, especially those bearing weight; also called *degenerative arthritis*.

Osteoarthropathy   Any disease involving bones and joints accompanied by pain.

Osteochondritis (os'te-o-kon-dri'tis)   Inflammation of bone and cartilage.

Osteoma   A bony tumour; also called *exostosis*.

Osteomyelitis (os-te-o-mi-el-i'-tis)   Inflammation of bone and marrow.

Osteotome (os'te-o-tom)   A surgical chisel, used to cut bone.

Osteotomy (os'te-ot'o-me)   Cutting through bone.

Osteotripsy   Rasping of a bone.

Pallor (pal'-or)   Paleness of the skin.

Papilloma (pap-il-lo'-mah)   An innocent growth of epithelial tissue; *see also* Verruca.

Papule (pap'-ule)   A small raised lesion up to a centimetre in size.

Paraesthesia/paresthesia (par-es-the'ze-ah)   *'Pins and needles'*, abnormal tingling sensation.

Paralysis   Muscle weakness that varies in its degree and extent of severity.

Parkinsonism   A disorder characterized by tremor, rigidity and poverty of spontaneous movement.

Paronychia (par-on-ik'-e-ah)   *'Whitlow'*, an inflammation of the medial or lateral nail folds.

Pedicle (ped'-ik-l)   The narrow stem of tissue connecting tumours to normal tissue.

Penrose tourniquet   A small tourniquet used around a digit.

Periosteum (per'e-os'te-um)   A layer of connective tissue that covers the surface of bone except at the articular surface.

Periostitis (per'e-os-ti'tis)   Inflammation of the periosteum.

Peroneal (per'o-ne'al)   Pertaining to the fibular side of the leg.

Peroneus (per'o-ne'us)   One of the peroneus muscles of the leg that arises from the fibula. The *peroneus longus* and *peroneus brevis* are situated at the side of the leg and inserted into the fifth metatarsal bone of the foot.

Pes cavus   An abnormally high longitudinal arch of the foot.

Pes planus (pla'nus)   *'Flat foot'*, an abnormally low longitudinal arch of the foot.

Phalangeal (fah-lan'je-al)   Pertaining to a phalanx.

Phalangectomy (fal'an-jek'to-me)   Surgical removal of a phalanx.

Phalanges (fal'an'-jez)   The bones of the toes.

Phalangitis (fal'an-ji'tis)   Inflammation of a phalanx.

Phalanx (fa'lanks)   Any bone of a toe.

Phenol   A chemical used in the destruction of the nail matrix; also called *carbolic acid*.

Phlebitis   Inflammation of a vein.

Pitting oedema/edema (e-de'mah)   The swelling of tissue due to an excessive accumulation of fluid in which fingertip pressure leaves temporary indentations in the skin.

Plantar   Pertaining to the sole of the foot.

Plantar arch   The arch in the sole of the foot formed by the plantar arteries.

Plantar fasciitis   Inflammation of the fascia on the sole of the foot.

Plantar reflex   A reflex obtained by drawing a blunt object along the lateral border of the sole of the foot from the heel to the little toe; the normal *flexor response* is a downward movement of the toes. An upward movement of the great toe is called an *extensor response* (the Babinski reflex). In all persons over the age of 18 months this is an indication of disease of the brain or spinal cord.

Plantar wart   A wart on the sole of the foot; medical name *verruca plantaris*.

Podarthritis (pod'ar-thri'tis)   Inflammation of the joints of the feet.

Polydactyly (pol'e-dak'ti-le)   The presence of supernumerary digits.

Posterior   Situated at or near the back.

Posterior tibial pulse   The pulse located on the medial aspect of the ankle, immediately posterior to the malleolus.

Povidone–iodine   A complex of iodine in an organic carrier medium, used as a topical antiseptic; trade name *Betadine*®.

Prilocaine   A local anaesthetic; trade name *Citanest*®.

Prophylactic   Pertaining to an agent that tends to ward off disease.

Prophylaxis   Any treatment taken to prevent infection or disease.

Prosthesis (pros-the'sis)   An artificial device that is attached to the body used for functional or cosmetic reasons.

Proximal   Situated close to the origin or point of attachment or close to the median line of the body.

Pruritus   Itching.

Psoriasis (so-ri'ah-sis)   A skin disease in which scaly red patches form on the elbows, knees and other parts of the body.

Pus (pus)   A thick greenish or yellowish liquid formed at the site of an established infection.

Pustule   A small elevation of skin containing pus.

Range of motion Within joints, the movement from one endpoint to another.

Rasp/raspatory (ras'pah-to-re) A file used for scraping the surface of bone; also called a *xyster*.

Reagent A substance used to produce a chemical reaction.

Reflex An involuntary response to a stimulus.

Resect (re-sekt) To excise a part of a structure or organ.

Retractor A surgical instrument used to expose the operation site by drawing aside the cut edges of a wound.

Rheumatism A term for a variety of acute and chronic disorders characterized by inflammation and stiffness of muscles and joints.

Ringworm (tinea) A fungus infection often found on the feet and nails.

Rongeur A forceps used for cutting small amounts of bone.

Rupture (rup'chur) A tearing apart of an organ or tissues.

Salicylic acid A chemical used in the treatment of verruca.

Saphenous Pertaining to or associated with the saphenous vein or nerve in the leg.

Scalpel Small, pointed surgical knife.

Sebaceous cyst (se-ba'shus) A cyst filled with sebum arising in a sebaceous gland of the skin.

Second intention Healing by granulation.

Sepsis (sep'sis) The destruction of tissue by disease-causing bacteria or their toxins.

Sequestrectomy (se'kwes-trect'o'me) The excision of a sequestrum.

Sequestrum (se'kwes'trum) A detached portion of dead bone.

Serous fluid (ser'us) Liquids of the body, similar to blood serum, that are in part secreted by serous membranes.

Sesamoid bone A small bone that lies within a tendon (under the head of the first metatarsal in the foot).

Sesamoidectomy Excision of a sesamoid bone.

Sesamoiditis Inflammation of a sesamoid bone.

Silver nitrate A chemical used in the treatment of verruca.

Sinus (si'nus) A tract leading from a focus of infection to the surface of the skin.

Slough (sluf) Tissue that separates from healthy tissue after inflammation or infection.

Sphygmomanometer (sfig-mo-man-om'e-ter) An instrument used to measure blood pressure in the arteries.

Sponge A sterile pad made of an absorbent material used in surgery; *see also* Gauze, Swab.

Spoon nail A toe nail having a concave surface.

Spring ligament Interior calcaneonavicular ligament of the foot.

Square knot A surgical double knot in which ends and standing parts are together and parallel to each other.

Sterile (ster'il) Free from living microorganisms.

Sterilization (ster'il-i-za'shun) The process of completely removing or destroying microorganisms by exposure to chemical or physical agents.

Stress fracture A fine hairline fracture that appears without evidence of soft tissue damage; it may not become visible on X-ray examination until 3 to 4 weeks after the onset of symptoms; also called *March fracture*.

Subcutaneous Beneath the skin.

Subcuticular Beneath the epidermis; also called *subepidermal*.

Subluxation Partial dislocation of a joint.

Subtalar joint The articulation of the talus and calcaneus.

Subungual (sub-ung'gwal) Under the nail.

Subungual haematoma/hematoma A collection of blood under the nail. May be treated by heating the end of a paper clip and then placing its point against the nail to melt a small hole so that the blood is permitted to escape.

Sulcus (sul'-kus) An infolding of the skin at the sides of nails.

Superficial Situated close to the surface.

Superficial reflex A reflex induced by a very light stimulus, such as stroking with cotton wool.

Superflexion Excess flexion.

Supinate (su'pi-nat) To rotate the foot and leg outward.

Supine (su'-pin)   Lying with the face upward.

Suture (su'-chur)   The thread or wire used in surgery for stitching tissue together.

Swab   See *sponge*; also cotton or gauze on the end of a slender stick used for cleaning cavities or taking bacteriological specimens.

Syncope (sin'-ku-pe)   *'Fainting'*, a temporary loss of consciousness caused by inadequate blood flow to the brain.

Syndactylism (sin-dak'-til-izm)   *'Webbing'*, congenital fusion of the toes.

Synovial membrane (si-no'-ve-al)   A serous membrane lining the articular capsule of a movable joint.

Synovitis (si-no-vi'-tis)   Inflammation of a synovial membrane.

Tachycardia (tak-e-kar'-de-ah)   An increase in the heart rate above normal; over 100 beats per minute.

Tailor's bunion   Enlargement of the lateral aspect of the fifth metatarsal head; also called *bunionette*.

Talus (ta'-lus)   The bone articulating with the tibia, fibula, calcaneus and navicular bone. The second largest bone in the foot.

Tarsal   Pertaining to the bones of the ankle and foot.

Tarsus   The seven bones of the proximal part of the foot.

Telangiectasis   A vascular lesion formed by dilatation of a small group of blood vessels. Frequently seen on the ankle.

Tendon   A tough whitish cord, consisting of bundles of collagen fibres, which serves to attach bone to muscle.

Tendonitis   Inflammation of a tendon.

Tenectomy   Excision of a tendon.

Tenoplasty   The plastic repair of a tendon.

Tenosynovitis   Inflammation of a tendon or a sheath of a tendon.

Tenotomy   The division of a tendon.

Thrombosis (throm-bo'-sis)   When a thrombus has become detached from its site of origin and carried in the blood to lodge in another part.

Thrombus (throm'-bus)   A stationary blood clot.

Tibia   The inner and larger bone of the lower leg.

Tinea pedis (tin'e-ah)   *'Athlete's foot'*, a fungus infection occurring on the foot.

Tourniquet (toor'-ni-ket)   Any constrictor used on an extremity to apply pressure over an artery to arrest bleeding.

Trauma   An injury or wound caused by external force or violence.

Trigger toe   An impairment in the ability to extend the toe.

Trocar (tro'kar)   A sharply pointed instrument contained in a cannula. Used for the aspiration of fluids.

Tubercle (tu'-ber-kl)   A small rounded protuberance on a bone.

Tuberosity (tu-ber-os'i-te)   A large protuberance on a bone.

Tumour/tumor (tu'-mor)   Any abnormal enlargement in or on part of the body, normally applied to a growth of tissue that may be benign or malignant.

Tylosis (ti-lo'sis)   The formation of callus on the skin.

Ulcer (ul'-ser)   A well-defined area of excavation into the skin or an organ, resulting from inflammation or ischaemia.

Ungual (ung'-gwal)   Pertaining to the nails.

Unguis (ung'-gwis)   Finger nail or toe nail.

Valgus (val'-gus)   Bending or twisting outwards from the midline, as in *hallux valgus*.

Varicose veins (var'i-kos)   Veins that are distended and tortuous with incompetent values. The saphenous veins of the legs are most commonly affected.

Varus (va'-rus)   Turned inwards, towards the midline.

Vascular (vas'-ku-lar)   Pertaining to or supplied with blood vessels.

Vasoconstrictor (vas'-o-kon-strik'tor)   An agent used to constrict a blood vessel such as adrenaline (epinephrine).

Vein   A blood vessel conveying blood towards the heart.

Venepuncture/venipuncture (ve-ne-punk'-ture)   The insertion of a needle into a vein usually to obtain a blood specimen.

Verruca   *'Wart'*, a small benign growth on the skin, caused by a papillomavirus.

Vesicle (ves'-ik-l)   A small blister containing fluid, smaller than a bulla.

Virulent (vir'-u-lent)   Malignant; poisonous. *Virulent infection*—one that is abnormally severe and dangerous.

Virus (vir-rus)   A minute living organism smaller than a bacterium.

Vitiligo (vit-il-i'-go)   A skin disease in which areas of skin lose their pigment and produce white patches; also called *leucoderma*.

Warfarin   An anticoagulant used in the treatment of venous thrombosis to reduce the risk of embolism.

Wart   *See* Verruca.

Whitlow (hwit-lo)   Suppurative inflammation of a toe, near the nail; medical name *paronychia*.

Zimmer (zim'-er)   A four-legged walking frame.

Bibliography and suggested further reading

Brigden R J 1988 Operating theatre technique, 5th edn. Churchill Livingstone, New York

Ford M J, Robertson C E, Munro J F 1990 Manual of medical procedures. Churchill Livingstone, New York

Kaczmarowski N 1982 Patient care in the operating room. Churchill Livingstone, New York

Kumar B 1990 Working in the operating department. Churchill Livingstone, New York.

Saleh M, Sodera V K 1988 Illustrated handbook of minor surgery and operative technique. Heinemann, Oxford

Wardrope J, Edhouse J A 1999 The management of wounds and burns, 2nd edn. Oxford University Press, Oxford

Index